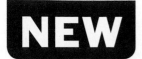

NEW

ANATOMY
FOR STRENGTH &
FITNESS TRAINING

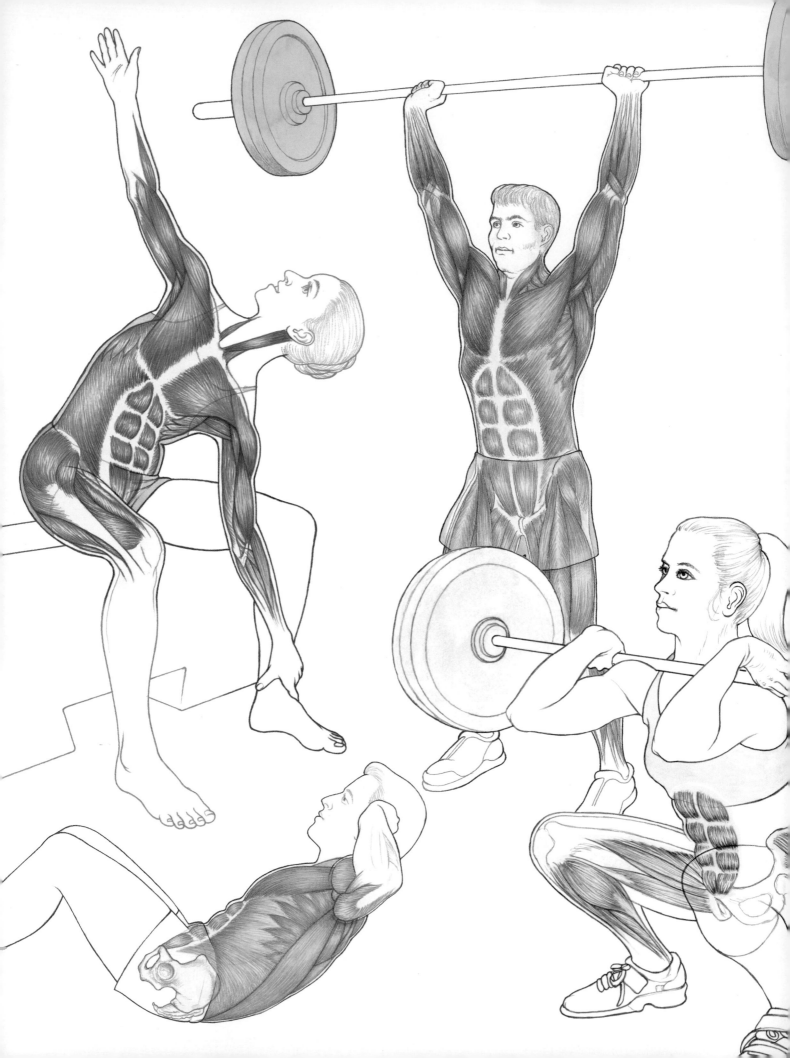

NEW ANATOMY FOR STRENGTH & FITNESS TRAINING

AN ILLUSTRATED GUIDE TO YOUR MUSCLES IN ACTION

INCLUDING EXERCISES USED IN CROSSFIT®, P90X®, AND OTHER POPULAR FITNESS PROGRAMS

MARK VELLA

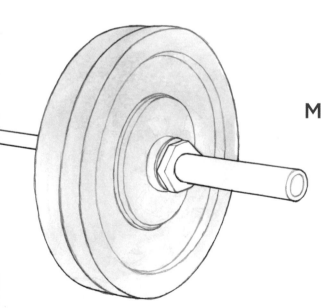

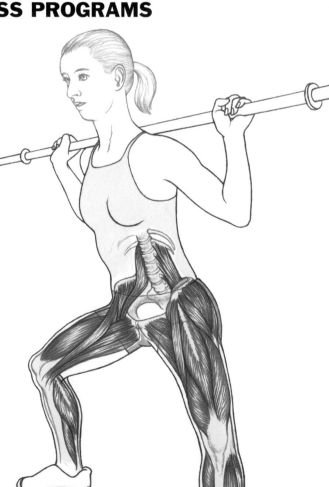

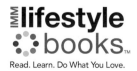
IMM lifestyle books™

Read. Learn. Do What You Love.

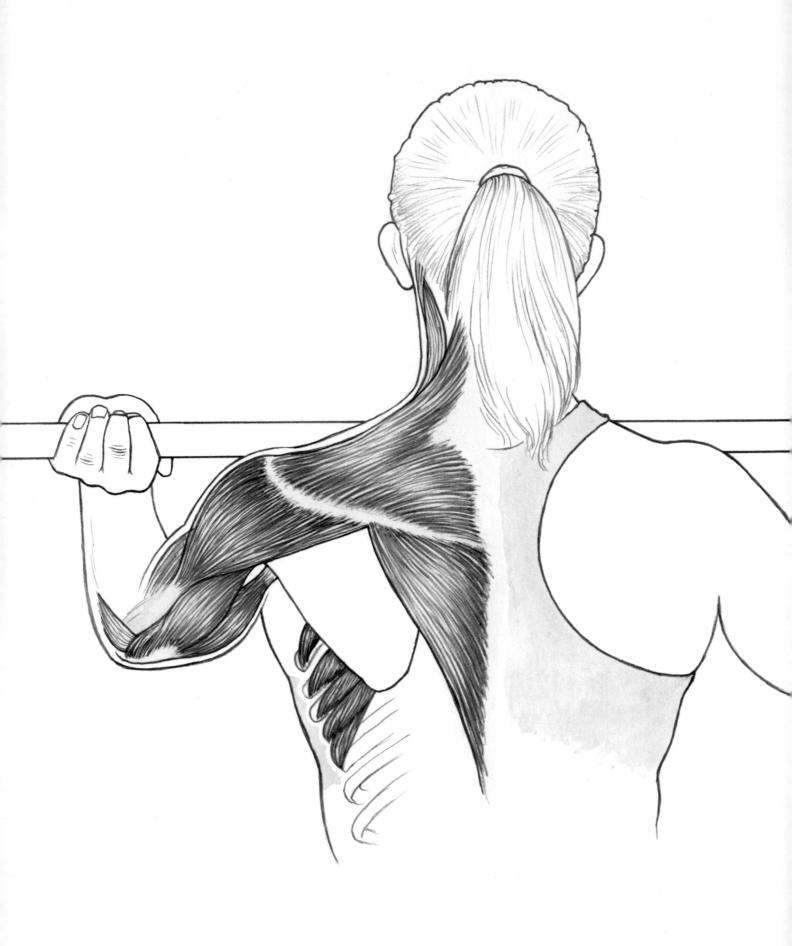

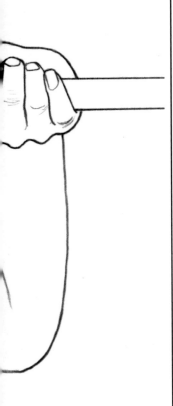

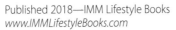

"There are anatomy books. There are exercise analysis and kinesiology books. There are exercise guidebooks. But never has there been a book that incorporates all three. This is that book. A fascinating and unique experience of the body."

—MARK VELLA

Published 2018—IMM Lifestyle Books
www.IMMLifestyleBooks.com

IMM Lifestyle Books are distributed by Fox Chapel Publishing, 903 Square Street, Mount Joy, PA 17552, *www.FoxChapelPublishing.com*.

Color illustrations by James Berrangé except on page 144 by Juliet Percival. Black and white illustrations by Evan Oberholster except on pages 59, 56, 64, 66, 68, 72, 74, 82, 95, 96, 99, 103, and 125 by James Berrangé and pages 12–13, 32, 33, 34, 35, 37, 38, 39, and 93 by Stephen Dew. Shutterstock photos: Kjetil Kolbjornsrud (page 20), Syda Productions (page 21 left), Tono Balaguer (page 21 right), David Tadevosian (page 22), Bojan Milinkov (page 23 top), LightField Studios (page 23 bottom), Antonia Giroux (page 24 top), antoniodiaz (page 24 bottom), wavebreakmedia (page 25).

Fitness reader: Hannah Giagnocavo

New Anatomy for Strength and Fitness Training is a collection of new and previously published material. Portions of this book have been reproduced from the following books: *Anatomy for Strength and Fitness Training* (978-1-84773-153-1, Mark Vella, 2006), *Anatomy for Strength and Fitness Training for Women* (978-1-84537-952-0, Mark Vella, 2008), *Anatomy for Strength and Fitness Training for Speed and Sport* (978-1-84773-543-0, Leigh Brandon, 2010), *Anatomy of Yoga for Posture and Health* (978-1-84773-466-2, Nicky Jenkins and Leigh Brandon, 2010).

ISBN 978-1-5048-0051-8

The Cataloging-in-Publication Data is on file with the Library of Congress.

We are always looking for talented authors. To submit an idea, please send a brief inquiry to acquisitions@foxchapelpublishing.com.

Printed in China
Sixth printing

CONTENTS

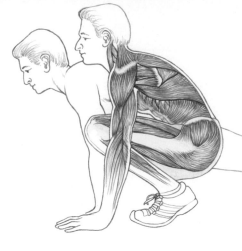

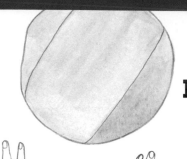

Foreword to the New Edition

When I wrote the original edition of *Anatomy for Strength and Fitness Training* in 2004, it was a hit, with close to 200,000 copies sold and translated into 9 languages. Since then, the world of fitness and exercise has been radically and beautifully disrupted and transformed by two forces: millennials and technology.

Whether you are a millennial or not, you may find yourself impacted and involved with many of the following exercise landscape changes.

If you are a millennial, born between 1980 and 2000, you make up a quarter of the US population, representing over $200 billion in annual buying power. In 10 years, you will comprise the majority of the economically active workforce. You have radically different values than your predecessors, Generation X. You have shuffled the cards on health and fitness and driven forward new trends through your non-traditional choices. You seek holistic, personalized workouts that are convenient, fun, and fueled by technology.

As a millennial, you have made fitness and wellbeing a bigger priority than any previous generation in post-war times. A 2013 report by the International Health, Racquet and Sportsclub Association states that 27% of millennials aged 21–30 belonged to a fitness club, a higher percentage than any other age group.

You are no longer content to simply accept marketing information driven through the mass media. In nutrition, this disruption is quite evident. Though you still want convenience and economy, as fans of low carb and Paleo eating, you seek organic, local, and artisanal food, and are prepared to pay more for it.

For you, holistic wellness takes precedence over more superficial values. You have eschewed the obsession over weight loss and challenged body image stereotypes. Quality of life, longevity, and feeling good take precedence over the obsession of looking good. Ultimately, you think of wellness as a lifestyle pursuit.

And so, instead of talking about work-life balance, you now talk of work-life integration. You look for working and living environments that embrace wellness as a norm. You take support from Google, coaches, and mentors for your self-empowerment.

As the first fully tech-savvy generation, you are fast-paced learners who like instant feedback and real-time measurement. You have adopted wearable technology like activity trackers and smart watches. You are more likely than any other generation to track your steps, heart rate, and caloric intake through these technologies and then use compatible apps to create personalized diet and exercise regimens.

As millennials, you have shifted spending from long-term assets to more meaningful, personalized lifestyle experiences. And this requirement for personalization, flexibility, and convenience can be seen in all aspects of your wellness lifestyle. Driven initially by Pilates and CrossFit, you began to seek out smaller group classes in smaller studios, closer to home or work, or even online, on-demand workouts from services such as Yoga Anytime or Zumba. You prefer exercise regimens that are individualized and varied to your needs, and, given your overscheduled life, that are shorter and more intense.

You have embraced the "gamification" of everything, from apps that gamify wellness goals to real life game-play in your exercise to increase the fun factor, such as obstacle racing like Tough Mudder or fun runs like The Color Run.

Even though steady-state cardio workouts may be the most effective way to lose weight, the traditional treadmill doesn't appeal to you. Because of this, you have flocked to workouts that continually vary and/or use high-intensity interval training (HIIT), such as Orangetheory, Zumba, SoulCycle, and CrossFit.

The Sports & Fitness Industry Association's recent annual report found that you are more likely to partake in physical activity that is more focused on community instead of competition. The cultures and fitness communities you support are reflected in your personal style and social media. This has driven the tribal group "#fitfam" culture as found at SoulCycle or CrossFit.

Given this radical change in the landscape, I was thrilled when I was asked to update this book. It was time to completely shift the book and its message toward a new, informed generation who embrace functional, multimode, compound training. Thank you to Colleen Dorsey and the team at Fox Chapel for embracing the new vision, and seeing the value in going beyond the original scope.

I have had the privilege of teaching movement anatomy for nearly 30 years now, having worked with close to 3,000 students and clients in the wellness and exercise domain. I thank all of you. May it never end.

My invitation to you, the reader, is simple: use this book. For entertainment, to be educated, and to empower yourself. Work with it. Refer to it. Let it inspire you to be a better you. Happier, stronger, and more positive, with something to contribute to this world.

Yours in health,

Dr. Mark Vella, ND (Naturopathic Doctor)
MAY 2017

DEDICATION

To you who made this book mean something in 2004 and now, may you always be peaceful warriors.
To Lynn, thank you for being by my side, in life and love. Every day with you is precious.
To Nuna, you are the beautiful full circle of my life. May you always have courage and be kind.

What's New in This Edition

There are many totally new exercises in this edition: Part 1 has undergone a complete overhaul, the glossary and resources in the back have been updated, and the content has moved away from gym and machine-based training, focusing on more compound, functional, and varied forms of training that are more current. We would have loved to include even more exercises in this volume, but there's only so much space in any book! It's our hope that you'll be inspired to find even more exercises that suit you after using this book.

How This Book Works

This book is a unique and exciting guide, reference, and graphic education tool in exercise and functionally oriented training anatomy. It is a visual and literal analysis of common exercises, as well as an exercise guidebook on how to do key exercises properly. It helps you to better understand the anatomy and the science of movement, known as structural kinesiology. Whether you are interested in understanding your own body and exercise program, or whether you are a coach, trainer, or teacher delving deeper into exercise science and anatomy, this book will give you many hours of fascination as well as a deep reserve of knowledge and personal value.

The book is divided into two distinct parts: Part 1, the primer, and Part 2, the exercises.

PART 1: CONDITIONING PRIMER introduces the gross anatomy of the musculoskeletal system and its movement and shares with you the relevant guiding concepts and training principles that can be used to develop and progress safely and effectively in training programs. It compares some of the new training options out there and offers some sample exercise workouts. It ends with an overall scaling map you can use to program your own workout or to scale an existing one up or down.

PART 2: EXERCISES comprises more than 100 exercises organized in 10 categories, including sections on stabilization, compound, plyometric and explosive, and endurance training exercises, as well as several body part sections, including chest, legs, hips, back, shoulders, and arms. Each of the 10 sections in Part 2 starts with a basic introduction that focuses on the body part or type of training. And each standalone exercise is a self-contained guide—you do not need to read the book in sequence! Each exercise includes several main features. The main exercise is defined and given some background at the top of the page. There is a starting position, description, and training tips section for each exercise, essentially comprising the "how-to" instructions for the exercise. There is a visual and technical muscle analysis of the main muscles being used, and you'll also find a color drawing accompanied by smaller start and finish position drawings.

NEW EXERCISE GRADING SYSTEM!

We have adopted a new color system in this book for quick and clear visual reference. **Green** refers to lower-intensity training and exercises suited to beginners/less-fit individuals. **Orange** indicates intermediate-level intensities. **Red** indicates advanced exercise for well-conditioned participants. You'll see this in the color indicators on the page corners and in the scaling guide (see page 26). Note that the colors are meant as a guide, not absolute gospel: exercises can be varied greatly just by changing speed, repetitions, resistance, and rest periods.

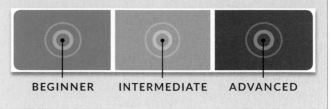

BEGINNER   INTERMEDIATE   ADVANCED

NOTE: There are more than 600 muscles and 200 bones in the adult human body. For the purpose of effectiveness and practicality, an emphasis is placed on around 70 main muscles involved in movement and stabilization. Many of the smaller muscles, the deep, small muscles of the spine, and most muscles of the hands and feet are not given specific attention. If they were, it might take several pages to analyze just one exercise and movement!

Waiver and Caution

This book is a useful tool, but it does not replace the expertise and wisdom of professionals who understand the art and science of conditioning, matched with the character that can support you, motivate you, and hold you back when you begin to overdo it. Seek them out and work with them.

DISCLAIMER

Many of the exercises in this book have a degree of risk of injury if done without adequate instruction and supervision. We recommend that you get a proper fitness assessment before undertaking any of the exercises, and that you seek qualified instruction if you are a total beginner. This book does not constitute medical advice, and the author and publisher cannot be held liable for any loss, injury, or inconvenience sustained by anyone using this book or the information contained in it.

Your Body: Quick Guide to the Musculoskeletal System

Your body comprises 12 distinct systems that continuously interact to control the multitude of complex functions of human biology. This book specifically illustrates and analyzes the muscular and skeletal systems, which control movement and posture. They're often referred to as one system, the musculoskeletal system. Interacting closely with these are the articular system (system of joints), the nervous system, and the more recently differentiated fascial system, which maintains the structural web of connective tissue on which the muscles are bundled and separated.

Movement anatomy has its own language derived from Latin and Greek roots. Knowing the language will help you make sense of the muscle analyses and terminology used in this book. If you are a student or practitioner, using the correct terminology will make your work more technically correct and precise and will facilitate technical interaction with other practitioners and work materials.

THE MUSCULAR SYSTEM
ANTERIOR VIEW

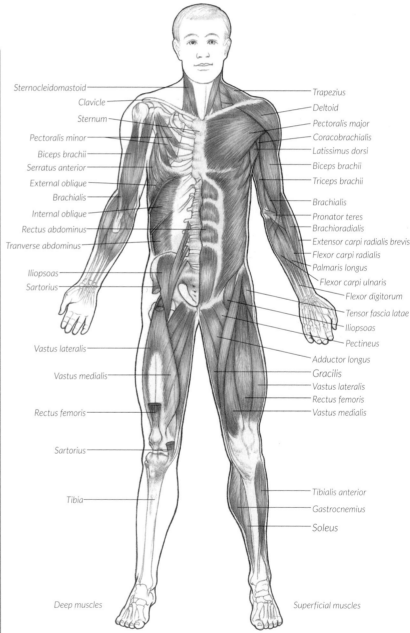

Sternocleidomastoid
Clavicle
Sternum
Pectoralis minor
Biceps brachii
Serratus anterior
External oblique
Brachialis
Internal oblique
Rectus abdominus
Tranverse abdominus
Iliopsoas
Sartorius
Vastus lateralis
Vastus medialis
Rectus femoris
Sartorius
Tibia

Trapezius
Deltoid
Pectoralis major
Coracobrachialis
Latissimus dorsi
Biceps brachii
Triceps brachii
Brachialis
Pronator teres
Brachioradialis
Extensor carpi radialis brevis
Flexor carpi radialis
Palmaris longus
Flexor carpi ulnaris
Flexor digitorum
Tensor fascia latae
Iliopsoas
Pectineus
Adductor longus
Gracilis
Vastus lateralis
Rectus femoris
Vastus medialis
Tibialis anterior
Gastrocnemius
Soleus

Deep muscles   Superficial muscles

THE SKELETAL SYSTEM
ANTERIOR VIEW

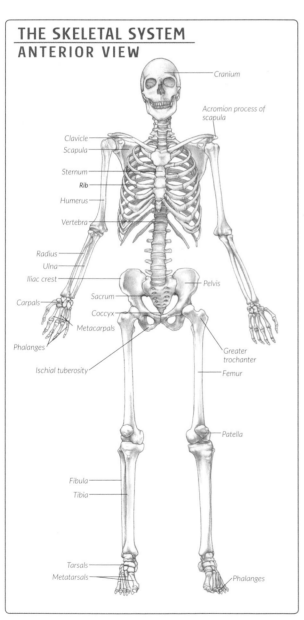

Cranium
Acromion process of scapula
Clavicle
Scapula
Sternum
Rib
Humerus
Vertebra
Radius
Ulna
Iliac crest
Carpals
Metacarpals
Phalanges
Ischial tuberosity
Pelvis
Sacrum
Coccyx
Greater trochanter
Femur
Patella
Fibula
Tibia
Tarsals
Metatarsals
Phalanges

THE MUSCULAR SYSTEM
POSTERIOR VIEW

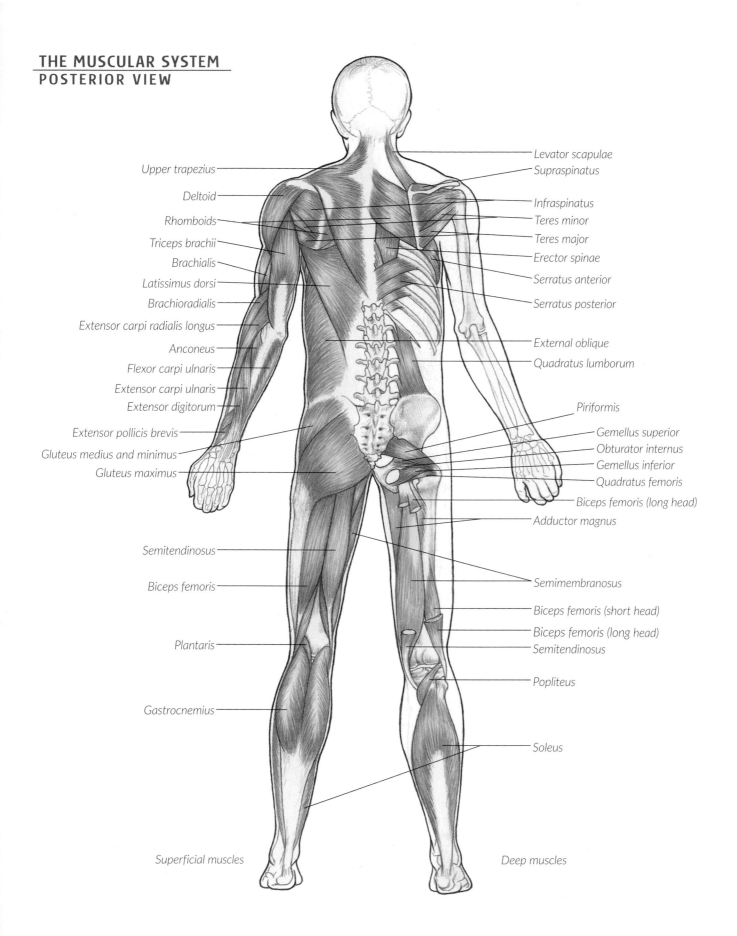

Upper trapezius

Deltoid

Rhomboids

Triceps brachii

Brachialis

Latissimus dorsi

Brachioradialis

Extensor carpi radialis longus

Anconeus

Flexor carpi ulnaris

Extensor carpi ulnaris

Extensor digitorum

Extensor pollicis brevis

Gluteus medius and minimus

Gluteus maximus

Semitendinosus

Biceps femoris

Plantaris

Gastrocnemius

Superficial muscles

Levator scapulae

Supraspinatus

Infraspinatus

Teres minor

Teres major

Erector spinae

Serratus anterior

Serratus posterior

External oblique

Quadratus lumborum

Piriformis

Gemellus superior

Obturator internus

Gemellus inferior

Quadratus femoris

Biceps femoris (long head)

Adductor magnus

Semimembranosus

Biceps femoris (short head)

Biceps femoris (long head)

Semitendinosus

Popliteus

Soleus

Deep muscles

Your Body: Quick Guide to Joints and Movements

Knowing and understanding the exercise movements, and at which joints they occur, is essential for being able to analyze an exercise. In this book, we have done the identification for you. In movement, while the articular system facilitates movement (initiated by the voluntary motor nerves), the skeletal system offers a series of levers upon which the muscles act, pulling on these levers at attachment points called insertions. When performing a movement, a combination of nerve stimulation and muscular contraction facilitates the movement that occurs at the synovial (free-moving joints). For example, when doing a bicep curl, the weight rises because the angle of the elbow joint closes,

Joint movements

The knee joint is the largest, the hip joint is the strongest, and the shoulder is potentially the most unstable joint in the body.

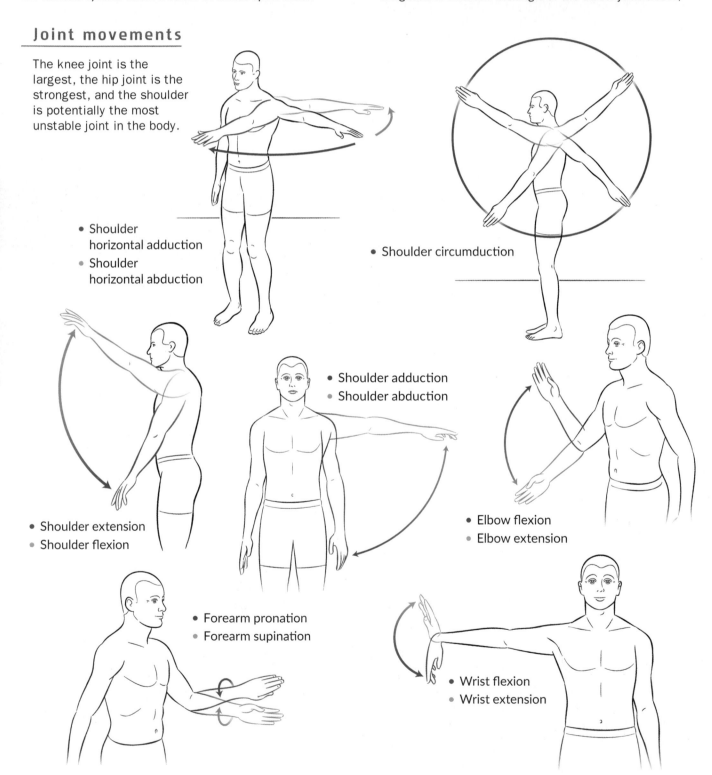

- Shoulder horizontal adduction
- Shoulder horizontal abduction

- Shoulder circumduction

- Shoulder extension
- Shoulder flexion

- Shoulder adduction
- Shoulder abduction

- Elbow flexion
- Elbow extension

- Forearm pronation
- Forearm supination

- Wrist flexion
- Wrist extension

as the bicep muscle, which is attached from the upper arm bones onto the radius and ulna, shortens in contraction, thereby lifting the forearm. Most joint movements are common names, applying to most major joints—for example, flexion and extension—but there are some movements that only occur at specific joints, such as ankle plantarflexion and dorsiflexion.

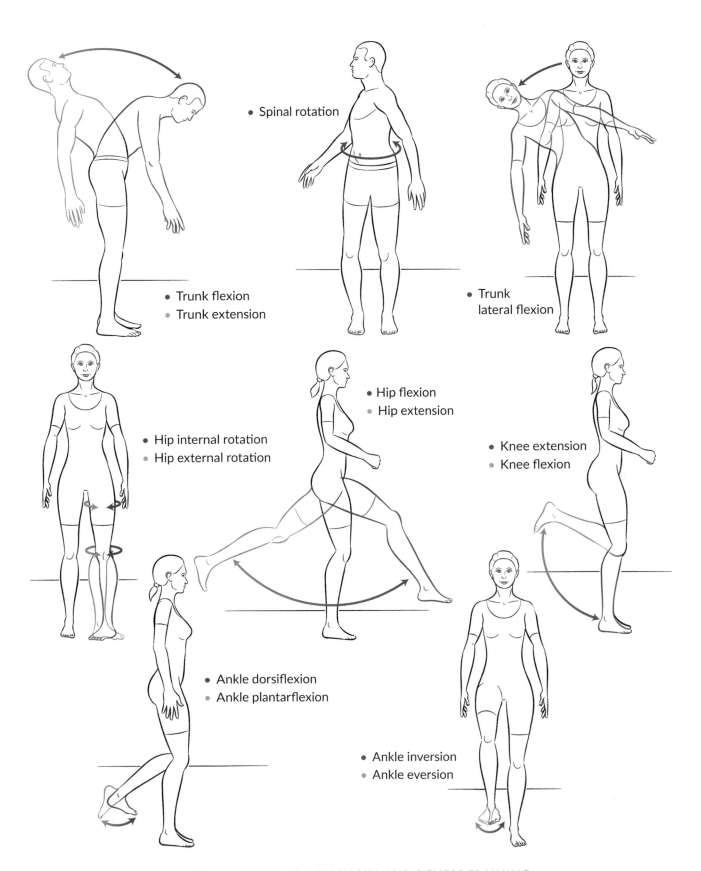

- Spinal rotation

- Trunk flexion
- Trunk extension

- Trunk lateral flexion

- Hip internal rotation
- Hip external rotation

- Hip flexion
- Hip extension

- Knee extension
- Knee flexion

- Ankle dorsiflexion
- Ankle plantarflexion

- Ankle inversion
- Ankle eversion

Training Concepts and Principles

WHY DO I NEED THIS SECTION?

I sometimes find that between all the academic information, journalistic license, and marketing-speak about exercise programs, people end up more confused, overwhelmed, and disempowered than ever before. Therefore, I felt it was important to clarify some of the current **concepts** and restate some of the principles that govern exercise programs, breaking it all down into simpler, relevant information that is easy for you to understand and use. Understanding these concepts and **principles** means you'll be able to see beyond fitness jargon, and you'll be more empowered to direct, progress, or scale back your training, avoid overtraining, and ensure that your fitness develops according to the personal goals you have set for yourself.

First, let's clarify the difference between a concept and a principle.

CONCEPT: This can be defined as a central idea. In exercise, it can be the basis or justification for a kind of workout. Because concepts are ideas, they are susceptible to human change and design. They come and go. Some are even old ideas repackaged as new ideas with new language. (This happens a lot in fitness, and in life in general). Some concepts, such as "core stabilization," drive long-term trends and behavioral change in exercise and fitness and form the basis for exercise types like Pilates or barre. Some concepts also appear as short-term fads that fade away as quickly as they appeared.

PRINCIPLE: This can be said to be a natural law that is universally applicable, with an evidence base in science (i.e., it has been proven), and that is true across a broad field of application, such as within exercise and fitness. These are laws that are best followed and worked with. Their consequences cannot be escaped. In our case, we are looking at the principles that apply to human exercise physiology, fitness, and how the body responds to exercise. Principles do not change. They apply no matter what ideas, trends, and fads are around. They apply whether you run marathons, do CrossFit, or simply exercise in your living room.

Here's a mantra I often use: understand and use concepts, but don't compromise principles.

IMPORTANT CONCEPTS

1. Individuality

Your current state of health and fitness is a product of four main factors: your genetics, history, lifestyle, and environment. The first two, for now, are beyond your control. The latter two are very much within your control, as you are able to make choices and changes around your present lifestyle and environment that can result in a more positive or negative expression of wellbeing. This is the power you have as an individual. Furthermore, even though our biological anatomy has all the same parts, we have a range of variability influenced by our genetic coding.

So, what's my point? Not every exercise program type, fitness program, or training protocol will work for everyone. Not everyone can start at the same level of intensity and exercise volume. Not everyone will progress at the same pace. This doesn't mean it's wrong or that you are weak; it just means that individual differences must be accounted for when starting and developing a training program.

There is no such thing as the perfect program. But I do believe we can say that there is such a thing as the perfect program for you, one that best suits your needs and goals. So choose a program that forms part of a healthy lifestyle and that is safe, effective, and rewarding for you, one that helps you be a better you, leaner, more mobile, and stronger in your own way. Start at a level you can maintain and progress from. Make time for your training. Get professional support, especially in the beginning, if you need it.

2. Physical Fitness

Before the Industrial Revolution, physical fitness was a product of an active lifestyle rich in manual work. Industrialization brought with it automation and sedentarism in a relatively short space of time. Biologically, our bodies had not evolved, but our lifestyles had changed drastically.

Into the 2000s, organizations like the American College of Sports Medicine began to define guidelines for health-related fitness, health promotion, and lifestyle disease prevention. As of 2012 reports, less than half of Americans meet the current activity guidelines. In fact, three quarters are regarded as sedentary. Around the year 2000, as the impact of millennials began to take effect, new opinions weighed in, defining physical fitness for a new, empowered millenial who is interested in pursuing greater physical attributes beyond just health promotion.

One the most current definitions of physical fitness, and certainly more apt for those interested in higher levels of performance, is that developed by Greg Glassman at CrossFit in the early 2000s. He defined physical fitness as increased work capacity and mastery of 10 main physical domains of functional fitness: cardiovascular and respiratory endurance, stamina, strength, flexibility, power, speed, coordination, agility, balance, and accuracy.

3. Functional Exercise

Functional training helps ensure optimum quality of life for everyday demands. It is a classification of exercise that involves training the body for the activities of daily living, in a way similar to day-to-day movement. This includes activities such as standing, throwing, lifting, pulling, climbing, running, and punching.

Functional movements use universal motor recruitment patterns. They are generally performed in a wave of contraction from core to periphery, and they are compound and multi-joint movements. A key principle in restoring and optimizing functional movement patterns is that postural stabilization should be enhanced first, along with full mobility of the body joint range of movements. Once that base is developed, higher levels of functional strength can be developed in the mobilizing muscles. Exercises used should be broad and varied, while being consistent in overload and frequency.

4. High-Intensity Interval Training

High-intensity interval training (HIIT) consists of repeated, short bursts of exercise, completed at a high level of intensity, followed by a predetermined time of rest or low-intensity activity. It is usually done in repeated cycles: for example, do as many reps as you can in 20 seconds, rest for 10 seconds, and repeat, repeat, repeat.

HIIT workouts are shorter and more challenging. The total duration of a HIIT workout can be 4 to 12 minutes, seldom 20. High-intensity workouts are generally considered to be 80% or more of your Predicted Maximum Heart Rate (PMHR) (see page 138). Recovery intervals are generally at 40% to 50% of PMHR to feel comfortable. HIIT protocols are widely applied to many kinds of exercise.

The recent popularity of HIIT stems from HIIT research protocols performed on a cycling ergometer by Japanese Olympic speed skaters using a format of eight cycles of 20 seconds of work followed by 10 seconds of rest. This became known as the Tabata protocol. This, and other research since, showed better results than more moderate, longer-duration programs. Additionally, many millennials feel they don't have the time for the longer, steady-state workouts. These workouts are therefore losing ground to HIIT-oriented workouts, such as Orangetheory, Zumba, SoulCycle, and CrossFit.

However, it's sometimes overlooked that true HIIT training can more easily result in injury and overtraining, especially in those without a fitness base and when overused. The truth is that most people who think they are doing HIIT workouts are probably doing more HIVT (high-intensity variable training). This means that there is much greater variation in heart rate levels and rest periods, thereby reducing the injury and overtraining component of the workouts.

PRINCIPLES WORTH FOLLOWING

1. SAID Principle

The principle of Specific Adaptation to Imposed Demands (SAID) says that your body will predictably change through an adaptive process in response to the exercise demands that are placed on it.

For example, if you begin running or jogging, the stimulus of running will result in an adaptive response in your body that will improve your physiology to become more suited to running. Basically, positive stimulus through adaptation leads to a better response. If you run regularly, you will become a better runner. If you cycle regularly, you will become a better cyclist. We sometimes also call this the principle of specificity.

How fast adaptation will occur is very much individually determined, but beginners or those in the lowest ranges of functional capacity are likely to improve the quickest.

2. Progressive Overload

To gain improvement in fitness, the body must be stimulated beyond its present capacity. So, for example, if you wish to gain strength, you must train with a weight stimulus that is higher than your present capacity. This amount of stimulus is called the overload.

To keep increasing our response in a particular domain like endurance, strength, or speed, we have to keep practicing. The principle of progressive overload says that this practice should be consistent, repetitive, and with a progressively increasing overload, to overcome the natural training plateau of adaptation.

There are 4 major variables of overload to any training plan or exercise prescription: frequency, intensity, type, and time/duration. To progress overload, one can increase training in any of these 4 major variables. However, progressive overload doesn't mean the training should be exactly the same workout every time, just with small increases. A degree of variety is fine and even necessary. That said, completely random and inconsistent programming may reduce progress in one specific area while creating more moderate gains in a range of areas.

If you decide to no longer keep progressing your overload, your training gains will plateau. And if

you stop training, your gains will reverse. This is the principle of reversibility.

When leveraging the principle of progressive overload, it is key that you perform the given exercise with good form and a stable posture. Progressive overload should never be prioritized over proper form. In turn, a base of strength is necessary before moving on to speed, power, and plyometric work. (See the Progression Pyramid below.)

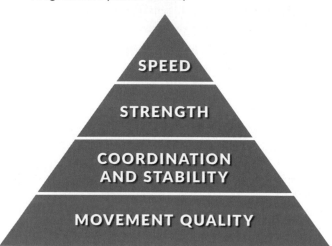

Progression Pyramid

3. Periodization

In the beginning of any fitness program using progressive overload, gains in fitness are significant for a beginner. Gradually, though, as we begin to reach our maximum potential capacity in that domain, fitness gains reduce in relation to the amount of progressive overload. This is a natural plateau. To offset this, intermediate and advanced athletes begin to plan their training into a more organized schedule of fluctuating cycles and periods, hence the term periodization. This allows progress to keep happening, even if in smaller increments.

4. Intensity

Simply put, intensity is a measure of how hard we are training in a given exercise or workout. When training at more moderate intensities, we can train for longer durations. When training at higher intensities, fatigue occurs more quickly.

As discussed in the previous section, shorter bouts of higher-intensity training yield good gains but also carry a higher risk of fatigue and injury if overused or used without a solid base of fitness.

Intensity can be increased in several main ways. In strength and power work, you could be lifting heavier weights, faster, and with more repetitions while shortening rest periods. In typical aerobic work, you could go faster at higher heart rates (see page 136 for a deeper explanation).

Simply put, the key is to train at an intensity that allows the progressive overload to keep making incremental gains in fitness capacity in the domain where we are striving for improvement. As the base for fitness improves and training plateaus begin to settle in, varying intensity is an essential part of a periodization plan.

> Make sure you have the mobility required to do any movement before you attempt to do that movement. Awareness of movement safety and proper form is useless if you are not physically capable of doing a movement.

CONCEPTS AND PRINCIPLES SUMMARY

- Take part in exercise activities that are safe, effective, and rewarding for you.

- Start at the right level and progress at a pace that is sustainable and gives results.

- Be consistent and progressively overload your training.

- Training will hurt somewhat. You will sweat. It will be uncomfortable. We call this good pain.

- It's possible to train too much, too soon, too hard, and with too little rest. Doing this will injure you.

- Pain is not the goal. Fitness is.

- Train functional compound exercises with variety.

- Do HIIT no more than twice a week.

- Vary your program, but not randomly and inconsistently—unless that's your training intention.

- As your fitness levels increase, bring in more variety and intensity with adequate rest to match.

- Consider setting higher long-term goals and developing a periodization plan in cycles to achieve those goals.

THE 3 PHASES OF YOUR FITNESS JOURNEY

Months 0–3

In the first 3 months, don't expect to always enjoy exercise. Being unfit is not fun to address. It's normal for your motivation to be relatively low and your resistance to exercise high at this stage. External motivation, like a trainer, can support you, but they won't do the work for you. If your training is effective, it's going to result in some sweat, good pain, and discomfort.

Once you make an exercise commitment, make it an appointment in your planner. Train three days a week at least, if you want results. Be consistent, be on time, and do the work.

Positive changes to look for at this stage are improved mood and better sleep. You may see some changes in your body, but avoid punishing yourself if you don't. At this stage, 75% of people drop off, so try to limit punishing self-talk—be your own best supporter.

In this stage, lay down the good habits around nurturing your being. By this I mean look after your day-to-day physiological state. If you allow yourself to get low, hungry, angry, or tired, your willpower is likely to fade, and you'll revert to old patterns of avoiding pain and seeking pleasure. Replenish your being with sleep, good nutrition, and healthy activity. It will give you energy, willpower, and the courage to take better action and break old patterns.

Months 3–12

You will begin to see real physical changes. Your body becomes training-adapted, and training becomes part of your habit and routine. People start noticing. At this stage, you can start working toward some goals, increasing your overload and variety. Discipline and effectiveness are key. Overdoing it at this stage will lead to burnout; getting lazy will regress your hard-earned momentum.

Months 12+

By this point, you have worked hard to change your body and your health. Motivation has become intrinsic and exercise is an established lifestyle habit. Bigger goals, competitions, and sports events can be used to motivate you. To offset a training plateau and to avoid falling into a rut, periodize and plan your training into cycles and patterns more while still keeping perspective on the rest of your lifestyle. Consider setting some larger long-term goals. This may also be a good time to consult with a specialist trainer to further individuate your training or acquire more technical information and skills.

Training Options

The range of exercise options available nowadays is mindboggling. There have never been more branded exercise regimens and diverse training options, each often claiming to be the best. The marketing language that accompanies these can also add to the confusion. So how do you choose? Assuming you are just starting out (and have no contraindications to starting an exercise routine), following are some worthwhile guidelines when selecting a new regimen, as well as a quick guide to some of the most popular regimens out there today.

VALID CRITERIA FOR A STARTING WORKOUT REGIMEN

- **It's safe and structured:** There is support, safety is considered, and exercise instructors have the skill, knowledge, and maturity to show you proper technique and to scale you from beginner to fitter levels while taking into account your own biomechanical limitations.

- **It's sustainable:** You can keep doing it over a long period of time. It will grow with you, and you will grow with it.

- **It's effective:** It gets you the kind of results you are looking for.

- **It's affordable:** You can sustainably keep paying for it over a long period of time.

- **It's convenient:** It's manageable in terms of fitting into your time, location, and lifestyle.

- **It's rewarding:** It makes you happy in terms of results and personal enjoyment.

As you consider your options, bear this in mind: do not train to punish yourself for being unfit and not your ideal self. Forget the idea of a "best" exercise. See beyond the marketing fads and gimmicks, and get into something you can maintain, that is safe and effective, and that will push you to be a better you.

COMMON EXERCISE REGIMENS

Since 2004 and the first edition of this book, training has moved away from gyms and machine training and into studios, focusing on functional, varied bodyweight-centered training. A whole bunch of branded regimens have appeared in the past years, some as short-term fads and some as longer-term trends. Gyms, in turn, have responded by offering some of these branded regimens within their facilities—for

COMMON EXERCISE OPTIONS AT A GLANCE

PROGRAM	IN A NUTSHELL	POSITIVES
CrossFit	Strength and conditioning system using constantly varied, high-intensity, functional movements	Strong culture, community and support, functional, widespread, informative website, physical and mental toughness
Zumba	Latin-inspired dance exercise	Fun and social, don't need to be a dancer, widely available, home and online options
Pilates	Core stabilization training	Effective, widely available, can do at home, teaching standards, precision of instruction, mat options
Yoga	Mind, body, and spirit whole-body workout	Most popular exercise form, widely availible, easy to start, wide range of health and fitness benefits, lower cost, portable, well researched
SoulCycle	Upbeat stationary cycle class	Community culture and identity, upbeat, motivational
TRX	Home training device	Portable, well made, versatile, product support
Barre	Ballet- and Pilates-inspired barre training	Safe, effective, community
P90X	High-intensity home training program	Convenient, community
Orangetheory	Studio group HIIT (high-intensity interval training)	Monitored feedback, group motivation, upbeat, structured

example, an indoor cycling studio, CrossFit box (gym), barre, yoga, or Pilates classes within the gym. Some gyms have even created their own generic versions of trademarked regimens under a different name.

See the chart above for a quick comparison of some of the more recent common and popular workout regimens you can choose from, and continue reading for more details about each program.

LEVELS SUITED			GROUP EXERCISE	HOME EXERCISE	PRICE RANGE	WEBSITES
			Yes	Yes, possible	$$$	www.crossfit.com
			Yes	Yes, possible	$$	www.zumba.com www.zumbafitnessgame.com
			Yes	Yes, matwork	$$-$$$	www.pilatesanytime.com
			Yes	Yes	$-$$	www.yogaanytime.com
			Yes	No	$$$	www.spinning.com www.soul-cycle.com www.flywheelsports.com www.cyclebar.com www.pelotoncycle.com
			Generally no	Yes	$$	www.trxtraining.com
			Yes	No	$$$	www.purebarre.com www.physique57.com www.barmethod.com www.barre3.com
			No	Yes	$$-$$$	www.beachbody.com
			Yes	No	$$-$$$	www.orangetheoryfitness.com

Check out the social media pages of these programs on Facebook and Instagram. Many also have extensive videos on YouTube. Many gyms will offer generic versions of these programs at differing levels of quality, and many gyms also offer a free trial class for you to test a program out. Prices vary from location to location and country to country. There are countless regimens, spinoffs, and generic versions of the above programs, as well as many other popular forms of exercise, that we could not cover here; for example, TangoLates, Cardio Kickboxing, Hooping, and pole dancing. Additionally, there are many traditional forms of exercise and sport still popular today, such as Tai Chi, soccer, volleyball, and basketball, all of which are worth considering. As always, if you are pregnant, have any illness or injury, or have any other conditions that might limit you in commencing an exercise program, seek professional support and advice. Remember, too, that calorie count and physiological response to exercise are also subject to variances due to age, gender, weight, fitness levels, lean mass, and a range of other factors.

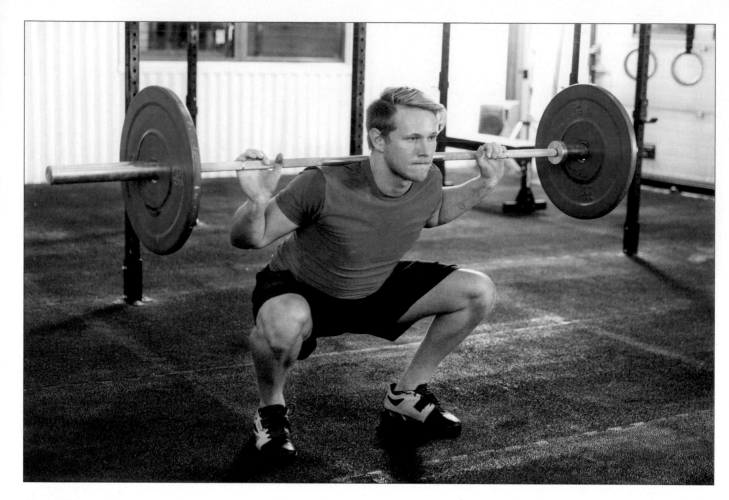

CrossFit

CrossFit is a system whose goal is to build strength and conditioning through constantly varied and challenging workouts. It is based on 3 principle tenets: exercise that is constantly varied, that is done at high intensity, and that uses functional movements.

CrossFit works almost exclusively with compound movements. Its exercises include Olympic lifting, powerlifting, gymnastics, strongman, girevoy (kettlebell sport) bodyweight training, plyometrics, indoor rowing, HIIT, running, and swimming. These exercises are combined into short, random, intense workouts that change daily, called Workouts of the Day, or WODs for short. WODs are usually done as fast as possible (called AFAP), or by completing as many reps as possible within a set time (called AMRAP). WODs are short and intense, usually between 8 and 30 minutes. Group classes are usually longer, up to 45 or 60 minutes.

CrossFit's philosophy is that everyone does the same WOD, whether they be a man, woman, old, young, well-conditioned, or not. Only the intensity (speed, rest periods) or load (weight, repetitions) is scaled.

It's hard to miss CrossFit's sometimes controversial and outspoken reputation for going against traditional exercise standards. CrossFit has been criticized on movement technique, high levels of intensity, and allowing under-qualified individuals to become CrossFit Trainers. To its credit, CrossFit has a loyal, passionate community, and arguably provides more coaching and support than in many gyms. It can be a humbling and encouraging environment that can build mental and physical hardiness. The competitive aspect can be motivating.

However, though CrossFit is open to everyone, it's not for everyone. The CrossFit method is intense. Overtraining is a common criticism of CrossFit. Another critique is its focus on speed at the expense of form: when doing AFAP or AMRAP, it's easy to let good form slip. Lack of a good coach spotting your form could exacerbate the problem. Beginners and those who are unfit, older, or who have physical limitations are at higher risk. CrossFit does emphasize teaching the basic movements until they are mastered before allowing participants to do the advanced lifts. A good instructor who has a solid foundation in conditioning and exercise is crucial to help you scale properly and to prevent you from overtraining.

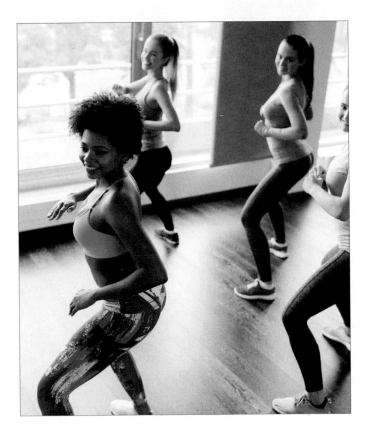

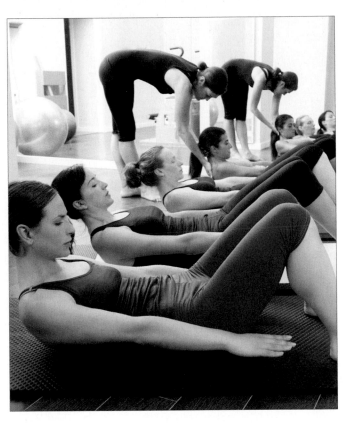

Zumba

Zumba is a regimen combining Latin dance music and dance moves in an energetic 45- to 60-minute class format. As a beginner, don't feel intimidated—there is room for your own interpretation of the dance moves. With its base in aerobic conditioning, Zumba includes elements of strength endurance, speed, flexibility, coordination, balance, and agility. It's a whole-body, moderate- to high-intensity class that burns 300 to 800 calories.

Zumba claims to be the largest branded fitness program in the world, with 15 million people doing Zumba in 200,000 locations in 180 countries worldwide. Zumba is highly social. You can find a local Zumba class via the website, or do a class at home using DVDs or downloadable apps.

Pilates

Pilates is a practice of mindful movement that focuses on strengthening core postural muscles and developing proper body alignment and flexibility. Today, two main philosophies of Pilates exist. Classical Pilates teaches the original method of founder Joseph Pilates, whereas Contemporary Pilates schools have developed the practice further while still maintaining the principles of Pilates. A third type, Clinical Pilates, is being used in rehabilitation, physical therapy, and other clinical areas.

If you try Pilates, a common starting point is group mat classes, which teach you principles and basic movements using slow, precise instruction. You'll also be introduced to Pilates' unique breathing patterns, which don't quite match the pattern of traditional exercise. Sessions typically run 60 minutes. You can also do mat work at home and use online classes from services such as Pilates Anytime.

With consistent practice, you can expect to strengthen your core postural muscles, developing pelvic stability and abdominal control as well as improving flexibility and day-to-day functional strength. Improved breathing, coordination, balance, and positive body awareness are benefits. Pilates is low impact. Weight loss and maximal strength (i.e., bulk and power) are not the focus.

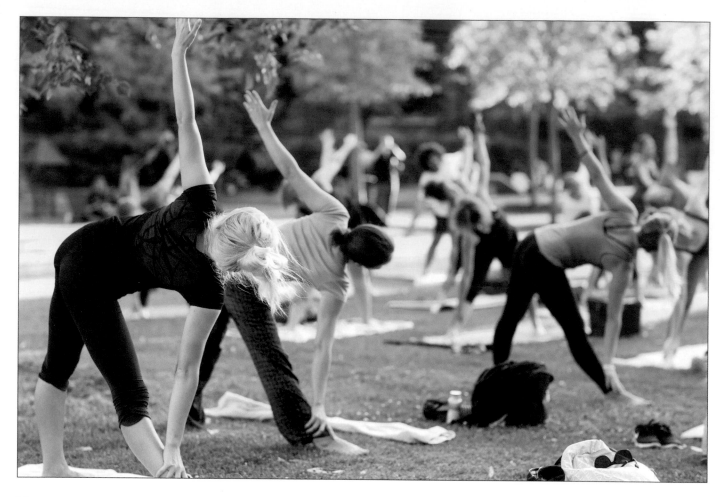

Yoga

Yoga had its beginning in northern India more than 5,000 years ago. The physical exercise aspect of the yoga lifestyle is called Hatha yoga, comprising exercise poses known as asanas. When doing Hatha yoga, you will go through a range of these asanas, in harmony with your breathing. Yoga is more than physical exercise—it emphasizes training your mind, training your body, and connecting with your spirit. Yoga can improve your flexibility, strength, balance, and stamina. Long-term practice has been shown to reduce anxiety and stress and to improve mental clarity and sleep.

Dress comfortably for your first yoga session. The average class is 75 to 90 minutes. You may find the strength, flexibility, and even endurance aspects challenging at first. Work at your own pace, with the teacher's guidance.

There are many variants of Hatha yoga for you to explore: fast-paced Ashtanga yoga and Vinyasa yoga, Bikram yoga (or hot yoga), spiritual Kundalini yoga, which includes chanting and meditation, and the precisely controlled Iyengar yoga, to name a few.

You can do yoga anywhere. At home, you can enjoy the motivation and instruction of online services such as Yoga Anytime as well as through countless apps. A basic yoga mat costs only $10. If you prefer group classes, they are plentiful and can range from a $5 student drop-in rate to $25 or more per group session.

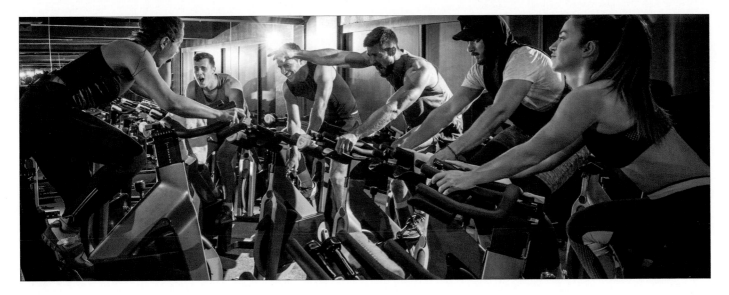

SoulCycle

Indoor cycling programs have spread worldwide, growing out of the Spinning workout and indoor bike developed by Johnny Goldberg in 1994. Of these programs, SoulCycle is one of the more popular, upmarket programs available.

In a standard 45-minute class, the instructor will lead you through a routine on a special stationary exercise bike with a weighted flywheel. Expect a candlelit setting, motivational coaching, and loud, upbeat music, with hand weights and upper body exercise included. There are also 60- and 90-minute workouts available. You can burn 200 to 700 calories per class.

Some find SoulCycle's cost steep and its atmosphere a bit cultish and loud. There are quite a few other indoor cycling options to consider, including CycleBar, Flywheel, and Peloton. The latter allows you to train through the Internet in the comfort of your own home.

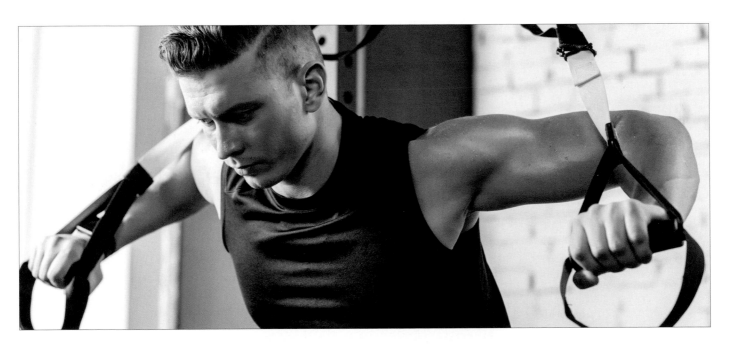

TRX

The TRX Suspension Trainer is a training device made from 12 ft (3.6m) of nylon webbing with handles and foot straps. Anchored to a doorframe, exercise machine, or other weight-bearing structure, it can be used at a gym and at home for a wide range of functionally oriented bodyweight exercises. Home kit versions start at $99. The TRX is cost effective when fully mastered. It is portable and versatile with quality construction. Exercise can be scaled on the TRX. It is largely suited to functional, compound, and bodyweight exercises.

Initially, the equipment can be awkward to use and difficult to master. This is especially true if you have poor core stability or a history of joint injury; these increase the risk associated with using the TRX.

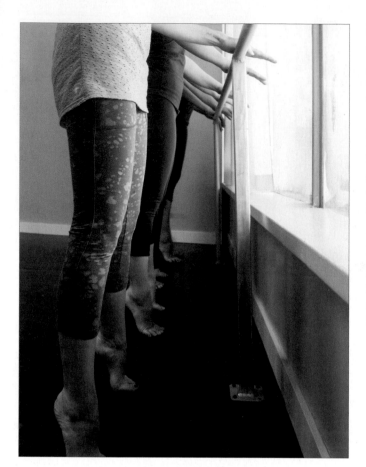

Barre

Barre is a total body workout that utilizes the ballet barre as balance tool to do mostly bodyweight exercises that are derived from ballet, yoga, and Pilates. In a typical barre class, you will start with a sequence of warm-ups and upper body exercises before moving to the barre, using your own bodyweight to focus on leg, hip, and core stabilizers, before ending in a cool-down stretching and recovery phase. The hour-long classes are intense, more advanced, and more strength-oriented than you may realize. Calorie expenditure is estimated to be 300 to 500 per class. Barre has a lower risk of injury, as it is mostly low impact.

There are several studio chains out there, including Pure Barre, Physique 57, The Bar Method, and Core Fusion. Most offer DVDs, equipment, and exercise apparel, in addition to online classes. Prices vary, though barre is more expensive than most classes. You may find it rigid and boring, especially if you do not have a background or interest in dance. In theory, it can be done at home, though this can be difficult without a barre.

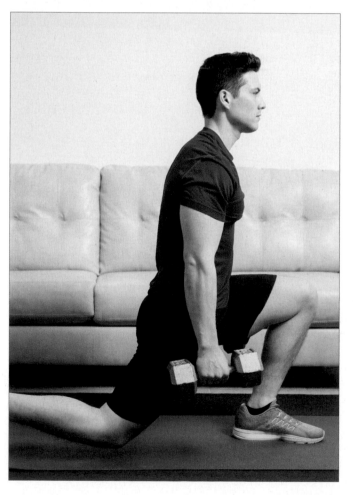

P90X

P90X is one of many branded home training programs delivered through online provider Beachbody, whose products include Insanity (HIIT cardio) and PiYo (Pilates yoga). P90X combines strength, endurance, yoga, plyometrics, and flexibility training, packaged as a 90-day DVD program comprising 12 workouts in undulating periodization cycles. Included with the program is a fitness test and a 3-phase nutrition and supplement plan. Workouts are 45 to 60 minutes a day, burning 400 to 700 calories, 6 days a week, and are for fitter individuals.

Aside from the $120 for the DVD program, you need to have yoga blocks and a mat, dumbbells, resistance bands, a pull-up/chin-up bar, push-up handles, a heart rate monitor, and a body fat tester.

Home training programs can be convenient, but they also lack group motivation. You may not enjoy the program's viral, social network-based marketing approach. If you are not fit, this program may be too much for you. Note that Beachbody coaches are devotees of the various online programs who have become salespeople through network marketing—they are not necessarily qualified trainers.

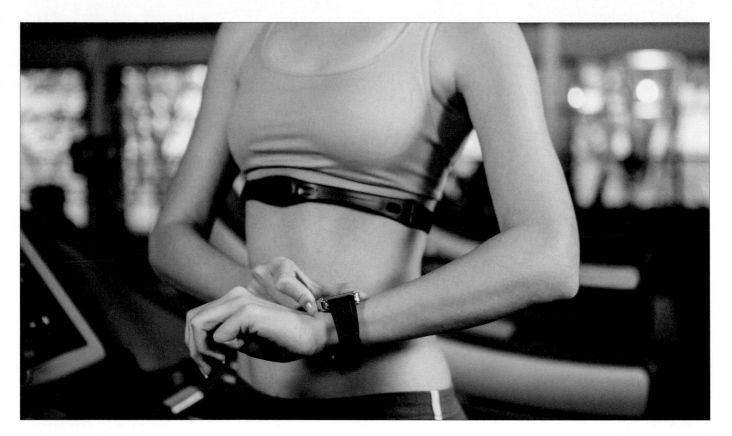

Orangetheory

Orangetheory studios offer 60-minute, trainer-led group workout classes of HIIT, blending strength, power, and endurance training. Treadmills, BOSU balls, rowing machines, and free weights are used in a circuit-style format in the class. As a participant, you'll wear a heart-rate monitor with your heart rate displayed on screens during the workout, providing you with real-time feedback on your performance.

Orangetheory workouts are based on the physiological concept of excess post-exercise oxygen consumption (EPOC). This refers to a state in which the body continues to burn calories at an elevated rate for up to 36 hours after exercise. Orangetheory achieves this by motivating you to work for 12 to 20 minutes in target HR zones, at a rate of 84% or higher of your maximum heart rate, thereby inducing EPOC. The class is designed to burn 500 or more calories per session.

Orangetheory studio fees are on month-to-month plans, but you can't use your own heart rate monitor—you must buy Orangetheory's. Orangetheory provides upbeat, motivating group training in a structured environment at prices similar to personal group training.

Scaling Guide

A scaling chart, also commonly called a training or movement hierarchy, is a way of representing progression of exercise choices based on movements. The scaling chart given here also serves as a roadmap of the main exercises in this book. While the color guides and individual pages help you understand each exercise in full, the scaling chart helps you understand where the exercises fit into the grand scheme of things. This chart specifically focuses on representing the exercise as it appears in this book and in the previous editions of this book. The chart is divided into four main movement tables, namely: Squat/Lift/Jump, Pull, Push, and Flex/Extend/Hinge.

The warm-ups, cool-downs, and technical skills training components of the workout are generally not included in the scaling chart. Neither are the aerobic/metabolic types of exercise, such as running or cycling. Nor does it illustrate the progression of overload by frequency, intensity, or time.

The scaling chart can guide you to know how you can regress or scale back an exercise if you are not coping and progress or scale up an exercise if it's getting too easy. Especially in the starting phase of an exercise program, you will be tempted to progress in overload too quickly; scaling back will allow you to get your technique and form right, allow your tissue biology to adapt to increased training loads, and mitigate against the risk of injury. As you develop, the scaling chart points the way forward in terms of progressing the intensity of exercise.

The scaling chart layout is not a perfect science, and there are several ways to arrange the movement hierarchy or classify exercises. A single chart cannot contain every exercise and each variation of every exercise. Bear in mind too that different types of exercise, such as Pilates, yoga, and CrossFit, will view the progression of exercise and even the types of exercise chosen through their own paradigm. However, some general principles do apply.

The four tables generally progress from left to right and from top to bottom. Horizontally, the most basic movements are on the left, progressing to more complex and explosive ones on the right. These more complex exercises are built upon the basic movements from the left. Vertically, the easier version of the basic movement will be on top, with progressions in technical difficulty, overload, and skill-related aspects of balance, coordination, and agility changing as you progress down the column. Wherever possible, you will tend to start with bodyweight movements and progress to greater overloads. You will also start with exercises with less technical complexity and establish a solid foundation in the basic movements. So as a beginner or less fit individual, you will start more on the left and top of a table and progress

through to the right and lower quadrant. Always default to the exercise that you can perform with good form. If you can't, or begin to fatigue prematurely, regress to a similar exercise or lighter load while maintaining enough overload stimulus to promote an adaptive response.

> **CAUTION:** *This scaling chart assumes a clearance for all exercise.*

BASIC WORKOUT STRUCTURE AND PROGRESSION

There are some general principles to follow when structuring a workout sequence. Review these four phases and try to design your own workouts to follow these guidelines.

- **Dynamic RAMP warm-up phase (6–8 minutes):** This is essential. It prepares your body's physiology for exercise and reduces injury risk. (See page 30.)

- **Skills training phase (10–15 minutes):** This is the best phase for quality of movement and technical learning. It can include form and technique work and stabilization training.

- **Main conditioning phase (8–30 minutes):** This is the main goal or theme of the workout. In CrossFit, this may be the WOD; in gym-based strength training, this may be your training routine for the day; and in aerobic training, such as Orangetheory or SoulCycle, this will be the conditioning phase in which you are working within your training heart rate zone. You will choose these from the four tables.

- **Cool-down phase (5–10):** Often ignored, this phase gives the body time to adjust its homeostasis and allows time for detailed passive joint stretching, relaxation, and meditation work, all of which contribute to the more holistic development of mind, body, and soul. (See page 144.)

To put things into greater context, beyond a single workout there is a systematic way in which to structure a workout program. Most exercise types will agree that a program that is varied, is done consistently, uses functional movements, and includes progressive increments in overload will result in increases in fitness parameters. As you look at the scaling chart, bear in mind that there are four ways to progress overload in any exercise. These four ways are:

1. **Frequency of training**

2. **Intensity via more weight, speed, repetitions, increased lever arm**

3. **Time or duration manipulation of exercise, such as found in HIIT, longer sets, shorter rest periods, etc.**

4. **Type, or progressing from one type of exercise to a harder type or version of that exercise**

In between workouts, the **rest phase** is equally important, allowing time for your body's natural catabolic and anabolic physiology to incrementally respond to the training overload, repair tissue, increase hypertrophy, and increase output for higher levels of performance.

KEY	
GREEN:	Beginner
ORANGE:	Intermediate
RED:	Advanced
ASFTW:	Anatomy for Strength and Fitness Training for Women, 2008
BB:	Barbell
DB:	Dumbbell

TABLE 1: SQUAT/LIFT/JUMP MOVEMENTS

	LEG SQUAT	LEG LUNGE	LEG LATERALS	JUMPS LEG POWER & PLYOMETRIC
	Squats with Ball between Legs (see page 70 ASFTW)	BB Lunge (see page 86)	Freestanding Lateral Lunge (see page 88)	Squat Push Press (see page 32)
	Bodyweight/Air Squat (see page 58)			
	Standing Squat (see page 55)	BB Reverse Lunge (see page 75 ASFTW)	Freestanding BB Plié Squats (see page 90)	Bench Step (see page 89)
	Back Squat (see page 60)			Standing Jump and Reach (see page 93)
	Front Squat (see page 62)			Wall Balls (see page 96)
	DB Front Squat (see page 63)			Box Jumps (see page 94)
				4-Point Burpee (see page 98)
	Overhead Squat (see page 64)			

TABLE 2: PULL MOVEMENTS

	PULL OBJECT VERTICAL, TO WAIST	PULL OBJECT FLOOR TO HIP	PULL OBJECT FLOOR TO SHOULDER	PULL OBJECT FLOOR TO OVERHEAD	PULL TO OBJECT
					Machine Cable Front Lat Pulldown (see page 112)
	Supported Bent-Over Row Machine (see page 100 ASFTW)	Modified BB Bent Leg Dead Lift (see page 78 ASFTW)			Standing Cable Pullover (see page 116)
	Seated Low Cable Pulley Rows (see page 120)	BB Bent Leg Dead Lift (see page 70)			Chin-Up Assist Machine (see page 96 ASFTW)
	BB Bent-Over Rows (see page 117)	Medicine Ball Clean (see page 72)			
		Sumo Dead Lift High Pull (see page 74)	Power Clean (see page 76)	Power Snatch (see page 78)	Bodyweight Chin-Ups (see page 114)

TABLE 3: PUSH MOVEMENTS

	PUSH AWAY FROM OBJECT HORIZONTAL	PUSH OBJECT AWAY HORIZONTAL	PUSH AWAY FROM OBJECT VERTICAL	PUSH OBJECT AWAY VERTICAL
	Wall Push-Ups on Bar (see page 58 ASFTW)			DB Seated Shoulder Press (see page 107 ASFTW)
	Bodyweight Modified Push-Ups (see page 104)			
	Push-Ups (see page 102)			
	Progressing Push-Ups (see page 103)	Bench Press Machine (see page 59 ASFTW)	Bodyweight Dips (see page 109)	BB Standing Shoulder Press (see page 66)
		BB Bench Press (see page 106)		
		DB Bench Press (see page 105)		
				Push Press (see page 68)
				Push Jerk (see page 68)

TABLE 4: FLEX/EXTEND/HINGE MOVEMENTS

	STABILIZATION	HIP AND TRUNK FLEXION	HIP AND TRUNK EXTENSION	KETTLEBELL EXTENSIONS	ARMS, FLEXION	ARMS, EXTENSION
	Posture Primer (see page 42)	Bodyweight Crunches (see page 52)	Double Leg Bridge with Shoulder Flexion (see page 50)	Bend and Reach (see page 34)	Standing BB Curl (see page 135)	
	Transverse Activation in 4-Point Kneeling (see page 46)		Ball Bridge (see page 51)			
	Abdominal Stabilization Program (see page 44)					
	Forward Stability Ball Roll (see page 47)	Bodyweight Sit-Ups (see page 53)	Alternate Arm and Leg Raises on Ball (see page 122)	Kettlebell Swing: Russian (see page 82)		DB Seated Overhead Tricep Extension on a Ball (see page 132)
			Back Extension Apparatus: Hip Extensions (see page 125)	Kettlebell Swing: American (see page 82)		BB Triceps Press (see page 134)
			Back Extension Apparatus: Back Extensions (see page 124)			Supine BB French Curl (see page 133)
			Prone Back Extension on Ball (see page 126)			
			Bent Leg Good Morning (see page 57)			
			Seesaw with Ball (see page 91)			
		Hanging Leg Raises (see page 54)				

Pre-Training Warm-Up

It's universally accepted that to warm up preceding an exercise workout is important, if not essential. Considering that this book focuses far more on functional compound training than its predecessors, a dynamic warm-up is not only critical to physical readiness for training, but is an essential aspect of mental readiness. It can also enhance performance and training results as well as mitigate against the risk of injury. A 2010 meta-study of 32 high-quality studies revealed that close to 80% of the studies showed improvements in performance following a warm-up.

DYNAMIC WARM-UPS

A dynamic warm-up generally consists of a minimum of 5 to 10 minutes of low- to moderate-level activity. It uses exercises and mobilizing stretches that move muscles and joints that will be used in the conditioning portion of the workout.

A **mobilizing stretch**, as the name suggests, involves the full range of movement around the joint. As it activates the muscle and joint through a full range of movement, it contributes to the neural activation requirements of warm-ups. A mobilizing stretch has been shown to improve performance after dynamic warm-ups.

Ballistic stretching, often unfairly maligned, is useful for elastic strength warm-ups and involves mild bouncing in the statically stretched position. Ballistic stretching is more advanced, higher risk, and should only be done by more experienced athletes as part of an extended warm-up. In general, mobilization stretching is the most functional.

In the past, it was not uncommon that **static stretches** formed the basis of a warm-up, together with some cycling or jogging. In a static stretch, a progressive stretch takes place in a static position. However, static stretching has not been shown to be of great value to pre-training warm-ups, and is better suited to the cool-down phase post-workout. Additionally, prolonged pre-exercise static stretching may well weaken the muscle about to be strength-trained—it has been shown to compromise subsequent performance, reducing power output, plyometric ability, running speed, reaction time, and strength endurance. The next time you see the 100-meter sprint at the Olympics, note how little static stretching the athletes do, and note how much ballistic and mobilization stretching they do.

In a dynamic warm-up, you can also include technique and form training as well as postural activation. This could be as long as half of the total workout time. This is common in CrossFit, for example, or other technique-dependent activities.

USING RAMP PRINCIPLES

RAMP is an acronym to describe a model and principles with which to construct a phased, effective warm-up. Developed by Ian Jeffreys in 2007, it provides for activation, mobilization, and potentiation of the muscles to be worked without developing undue fatigue. It helps you approach a warm-up with focus and purpose. The RAMP acronym stands for:

- **R**aise body temperature
- **A**ctivate the most important muscles
- **M**obilize your joints
- **P**otentiate the main muscles that you are going to use during that particular session

The RAMP acronym is apt. Think of an on-ramp to a highway. If you are traveling in a car, the on-ramp gives you time to bring your vehicle up to the speed of the traffic on the highway. The faster the traffic on the highway, the longer your on-ramp should be. Likewise, in your training, your warm-up should be longer if the intensity of the conditioning phase of your workout is going to be high, especially in training zones above 80% PMHR. If you have high levels of fitness, you'll typically also need a longer warm-up period.

Phase 1: Raise

The aim of the "raise" phase is to increase body temperature, heart and respiration rate, blood flow, and joint viscosity. It may include low-intensity, multidirectional movements or dynamic range of motion exercises.

Begin with low-intensity work. Assuming there are no health limitations, as you go through the RAMP phases, you'll gradually increase intensity through the training heart rate zones. For more information on these zones, see page 137. As you warm up, you should slowly and gradually increase your movement speed until you reach speeds and overloads close to that of the workout you are about to do.

Phases 2 and 3: Activate and Mobilize

The aim of this phase of the warm-up is both to activate key muscle groups and to mobilize key joints and ranges of motion to be used in the exercise. These can include doing lunging, squatting, pushing, pulling, and rotating movements. You can look at the fundamental movements and demands of your workout to come and then choose specific exercises and warm-up movements that mimic this. For example, if the conditioning phase of your workout is running, then jogging would be appropriate for the warm-up. If you're going to be doing heavy squat work, then air squats may be appropriate. Heavy bench press? Do push-ups.

Use full range of motion (ROM) movement to lubricate the synovial joint capsules, stimulate circulation, and warm up the myofascial.

Use accessories, where relevant. These can include foam rollers, skipping, battle ropes, medicine balls and ball drills, BOSU ball, kettlebells, and universal bars. The foam rollers can provide a form of massage to release tight areas and improve local circulation.

Postural activation is important. Given that you may come to your exercise session having spent much of the day sedentary, take time to center your awareness within your body through your breath. Pay attention to where you feel tension; focus on lengthening the spine, releasing joints, and activating your postural core in readiness for providing a stable and aligned base for the exercises to come.

Work through the planes. It's easy to only focus on forward-backward movements (e.g., cycling or jogging is in the forward-backward plane). Warm up your rotation, lateral, and cross-body aspects, too. Start with slow, controlled movements and gradually progress to challenging, fast-paced, multidirectional movement patterns.

The point is to gradually increase the intensity from resting levels to the intensity you have planned for the conditioning phase.

Phase 4: Potentiate

The aim of this phase is to prime, or activate, the muscles for the workout session. In this phase, the intensity will increase to the level at which you are about to work out. Therefore, this phase will see higher-intensity drills that are highly specific to the exercise to come. This can include sprints, plyometric jumps, and agility drills. If you are about to do intense compound functional weight training, you will simply choose the same base exercise at lower weights and higher speeds. As you move through this phase, weight and speed will moderate to the starting levels of the workout.

PHYSIOLOGICAL BENEFITS OF WARM-UPS

Circulatory Effects

Dynamic warm-ups increase circulation through increased heart rate and capillary dilation and decreased viscosity of the blood. This moves the oxygen- and nutrient-rich blood to the involved muscles at a greater volume, speed, and rate. Once there, the warm-up encourages the dissociation of oxygen from hemoglobin in the blood, improving the oxygen supply to the working muscle.

Hormonal Effects

A dynamic warm-up elevates your levels of hormones and neurotransmitters (such as adrenaline) that are responsible for facilitating energy production for the workout.

Joint Effects

Freely movable joints are encapsulated in a synovial membrane that is stimulated by movement to lubricate the joint surfaces. The movement of a dynamic warm-up stimulates the synovial membranes to release synovium, which nourishes the joints, reducing wear and tear and joint friction.

Neural Effects

Overall, a dynamic warm-up activates the nervous system, readying it for exercise. It increases the speed of nerve impulse conduction. Close to the joints, the adjacent ligaments that join bone to bone contain various sensory receptors that measure and identify pressure, movement, and rate of movement of their respective joints. The movements of a dynamic warm-up activate the regulating sensory nerve receptors around each joint, improving the stabilization and movement facilitation response. Warm-ups turn on the sensory receptors of the central nervous system responsible for identifying position changes in the body, which is essential for determining the appropriate motor response.

Myofascial Effects

Skeletal muscles are a combination of two things: muscle tissue proteins, and connective tissue and fascia that contain and separate the muscle structures. A dynamic warm-up elevates tissue temperature, decreasing the muscle viscosity. There is greater extensibility and elasticity of muscle fibers. The result is that muscles can more rapidly lengthen and return to their starting shape.

The muscle and connective tissues contain sensory receptors that sense tension, length change, and rate of length change. A dynamic warm-up activates these, improving their control of the muscle throughout the workout. This can then facilitate increased force and speed of contraction.

Overall, dynamic movement also increases body temperature, which increases circulation and makes the muscle and fascia more pliable, capable of lengthening and shortening at faster rates of speed. Think of how a ball of putty becomes warmer and easier to knead when you continually knead it in your hands.

The Result

As a result of all of these physiological responses to a dynamic warm-up, you will have the following at the beginning of the conditioning phase of your workout:

- **Faster muscle contraction and relaxation of both agonist and antagonist muscles**
- **Improved rate of force development**
- **Increased reaction time**
- **Increased muscle strength and power**
- **Increased viscosity, blood, and myofascia**
- **Increased oxygen delivery and extraction**
- **Increased blood flow to active muscles**
- **Increased metabolic function**

SQUAT PUSH PRESS

Dynamic/mobilization • Compound/multi-joint
Close chain • Bodyweight • Beginner to advanced

This exercise is not only an excellent whole-body warm-up, but it can also entrain the quality form for wall balls (see page 96), medicine ball clean (see page 72), and other medicine ball and compound, close chain work.

DESCRIPTION

Inhale, then as you exhale, squat down into a full or partial squat position. Without pausing at the bottom, return back to the start position while inhaling. As you return to the standing position, you push the medicine ball overhead. As you squat back down, return the medicine ball to the position at the chest.

STARTING POSITION

- Stand upright holding a medicine ball (5%–10% of body weight) against your chest.

TRAINING TIPS

- Keep the torso upright, eyes looking straight ahead.
- Keep the knees tracking over the second toes.
- Gently draw the umbilicus toward the spine.

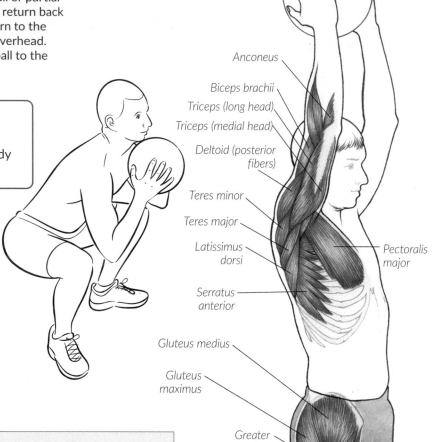

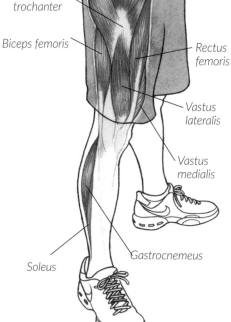

Anconeus
Biceps brachii
Triceps (long head)
Triceps (medial head)
Deltoid (posterior fibers)
Teres minor
Teres major
Latissimus dorsi
Serratus anterior
Gluteus medius
Gluteus maximus
Greater trochanter
Biceps femoris
Pectoralis major
Rectus femoris
Vastus lateralis
Vastus medialis
Gastrocnemeus
Soleus

ANALYSIS OF MOVEMENT	Joints	Joint movement	Mobilizing muscles
JOINT 1	Elbows	Up: extension Down: flexion	Triceps brachii, Anconeus
JOINT 2	Shoulder	Up: flexion Down: extension	Anterior deltoid, Pectoralis major (clavicular aspect), Biceps brachii, Coracobrachialis
JOINT 3	Scapula	Up: upward rotation, abduction (protraction) Down: downward rotation, adduction (retraction)	Trapezius, Pectoralis minor, Serratus anterior
JOINT 4	Hip	Up: extension Down: flexion	Gluteus maximus, Gluteus medius, Biceps femoris, Semitendinosus, Semimembranosus, Adductor magnus (posterior fibers)
JOINT 5	Knee	Up: extension Down: flexion	Quadricep group
JOINT 6	Ankle	Up: plantarflexion Down: dorsiflexion	Gastrocnemius, Soleus, Plantaris, Tibialis posterior

STANDING TORSO ROTATIONS

Dynamic/mobilization • Compound/multi-joint
Close chain • Bodyweight • Beginner to advanced

Use the ball to rotate the torso, not the other way around, in this warm-up exercise. This can also be done back-to-back with a partner.

DESCRIPTION
Rotate the torso gently in each direction. As you warm up, you can increase the range of motion and the speed. Begin by keeping the feet still. As you warm up, allow the feet to roll inwards as you rotate. The head can either stay looking forwards or it can rotate with the spine. Complete 10 to 30 rotations in each direction. Alter the height of the medicine ball to warm up different areas of the back and torso.

STARTING POSITION
- Stand up straight with a medicine ball just above the navel.
- Feet should be shoulder-width apart.

TRAINING TIPS
- Keep an upright posture, chest up and chin tucked in.
- Don't rotate too far or too quickly before you have warmed up sufficiently.

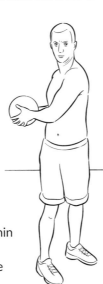

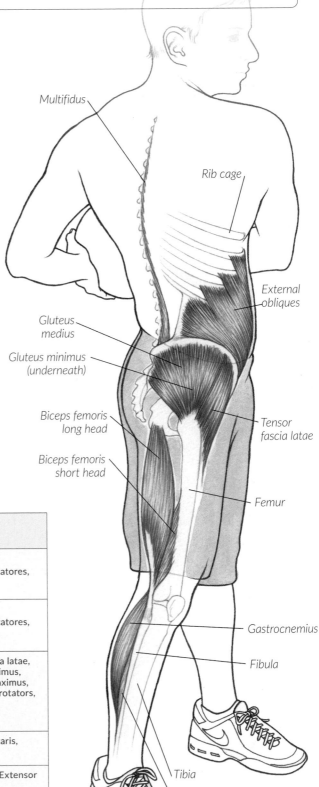

Multifidus

Rib cage

External obliques

Gluteus medius

Gluteus minimus (underneath)

Biceps femoris long head

Biceps femoris short head

Tensor fascia latae

Femur

Gastrocnemius

Fibula

Tibia

Soleus

ANALYSIS OF MOVEMENT	Joints	Joint movement	Mobilizing muscles
JOINT 1	Thoracic spine	Rotation	Ipsilateral: Internal oblique Contralateral: Multifidus, Rotatores, External oblique
JOINT 2	Lumbar spine	Rotation	Ipsilateral: Internal oblique Contralateral: Multifidus, Rotatores, External oblique
JOINT 3	Hip	Medial rotation, lateral rotation	Adductor group, Tensor fascia latae, Gluteus medius, Gluteus minimus, Hamstring group, Gluteus maximus, Sartorius, Deep external hip rotators, Iliopsoas
JOINT 4	Ankle	Plantarflexion	Gastrocnemius, Soleus, Plantaris, Tibialis posterior
JOINT 5	Metatarsals	Eversion	Peroneus longus and brevis, Extensor digitorum longus

BEND AND REACH

Dynamic/mobilization • Compound/multi-joint
Close chain • Bodyweight • Beginner to advanced

An excellent warm-up for the kettlebell swing (see page 82) and other compound, multi-joint work.

DESCRIPTION

Inhale, then exhale as you bend forwards until the medicine ball goes between your legs while keeping the chest up and eyes looking straight ahead. Inhale again as you reach up: the medicine ball goes overhead and you drive your hips forward. Without a pause, exhale as you return to the bent-forwards position with the medicine ball ending up between the legs. Complete for 10–20 repetitions, starting slowly and increasing your speed and range of motion as you warm up.

STARTING POSITION

- Stand upright with a medicine ball (5%–10% of body weight) at arms length in front of your pelvis.

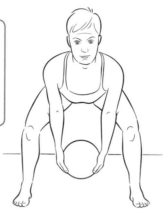

TRAINING TIPS

- Keep the torso upright, eyes looking straight ahead.
- Keep the knees tracking over the second toes.
- Gently draw the umbilicus toward the spine.

ANALYSIS OF MOVEMENT	Joints	Joint movement	Mobilizing muscles
JOINT 1	Shoulder	Up: flexion Down: extension	Anterior deltoid, Pectoralis major (clavicular aspect), Biceps brachii, Coracobrachialis
JOINT 2	Scapula	Up: upward rotation, abduction (protraction) Down: downward rotation, adduction (retraction)	Trapezius, Pectoralis minor, Serratus anterior
JOINT 3	Thoracic spine	Up: extension Down: flexion to neutral	Spinalis, Longissimus, Iliocostalis, Multifidus, Rotatores
JOINT 4	Lumbar spine	Up: extension Down: flexion to neutral	Spinalis, Longissimus, Iliocostalis, Multifidus, Rotatores, Intertransversarii, Interspinalis
JOINT 5	Hip	Up: extension Down: flexion	Gluteus maximus, Gluteus medius, Hamstring group
JOINT 6	Knee	Up: extension Down: flexion	Vastus medialis, Vastus intermedius, Vastus lateralis, Rectus femoris
JOINT 7	Ankle	Up: plantarflexion Down: dorsiflexion	Gastrocnemius, Soleus, Plantaris, Tibialis posterior

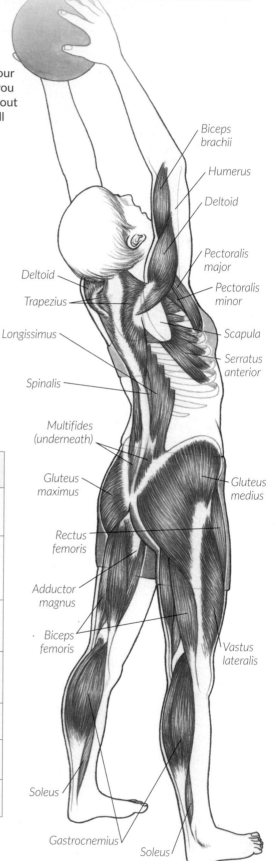

Biceps brachii

Humerus

Deltoid

Pectoralis major

Deltoid

Pectoralis minor

Trapezius

Scapula

Longissimus

Serratus anterior

Spinalis

Multifides (underneath)

Gluteus maximus

Gluteus medius

Rectus femoris

Adductor magnus

Biceps femoris

Vastus lateralis

Soleus

Gastrocnemius

Soleus

MULTIDIRECTIONAL LUNGES
Dynamic/mobilization • Compound/multi-joint
Bodyweight • Beginner to advanced

For all squat work, lunges, and hip work, this is an excellent mobilization warm-up.

DESCRIPTION
Lunge forwards and then back. Lunge forwards at a 45° angle, keeping the torso and feet pointing straight ahead and back. Lunge to the side, keeping the torso and feet pointing straight ahead and back. Lunge backwards at a 45° angle, keeping the torso and feet pointing straight ahead and back. Lunge backwards and back to the start.

TRAINING TIPS
- Ensure the knee stays tracking over the second toe.
- Keep the torso upright.
- Keep the torso and feet pointing straight ahead.

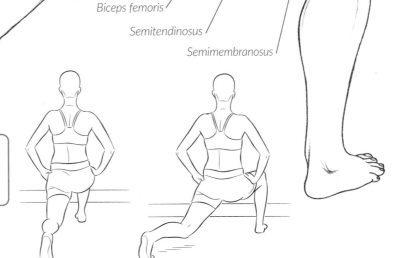

Gluteus maximus

Gluteus medius

Vastus lateralis

Pubic arch

Adductor magnus

Biceps femoris

Semitendinosus

Semimembranosus

STARTING POSITION
- Stand with feet shoulder-width apart and torso upright, hands on hips.

ANALYSIS OF MOVEMENT	Joints	Mobilizing muscles
JOINT 1	Hip	Gluteus medius and minimus, Hamstring group, Adductor group, Tensor fascia latae, Iliopsoas, Deep external rotators of the hip
JOINT 2	Knee	Quadricep group, Hamstring group
JOINT 3	Ankle	Tibialis anterior, Extensor digitorum longus, Extensor hallucis longus, Peroneus longus and brevis

SEATED STRIDE INTO SAW STRETCH

Static • Isolation • Bodyweight • Beginner to advanced

This is another total body stretch, this time focused on the lower body.

DESCRIPTION

Sit tall on your sitting bones with your legs flat at a 60° angle apart. Hold your arms horizontally with your chest open. Twisting your upper body from the waist, let your arms turn with your chest. Exhale, reaching your arms and trunk forwards and down toward one leg so that the opposite hand touches your inside lower leg. Hold the stretch at 4–7 on a scale of 1–10. Return, and then repeat on the opposite side.

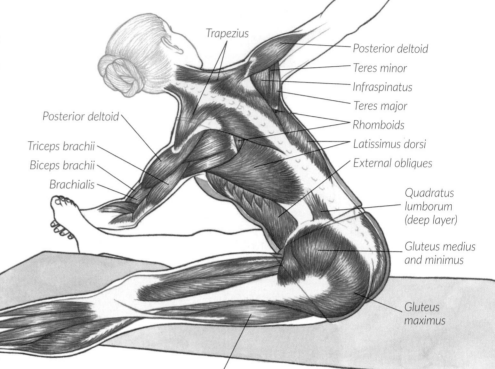

Trapezius
Posterior deltoid
Teres minor
Infraspinatus
Teres major
Rhomboids
Latissimus dorsi
External obliques
Quadratus lumborum (deep layer)
Gluteus medius and minimus
Gluteus maximus

Posterior deltoid
Triceps brachii
Biceps brachii
Brachialis

Biceps femoris

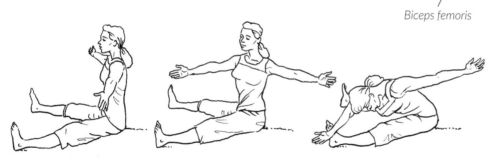

TRAINING TIPS

- Avoid forcing the stretch. Relax into it.
- Breathe in a relaxed manner.
- Avoid hunching or rounding your shoulders. Keep your chest open, shoulders relaxed and shoulder blades depressed.
- If your hips are too tight, modify the exercise by sitting on a small cushion or folded towel.

ANALYSIS OF MOVEMENT	JOINT 1	JOINT 2	JOINT 3
Active joints	Hips	Spine	Scapula
Joint position	Flexed and abducted	Rotated	Abducted (protracted)
Main stretching muscles	In both legs: Gluteus maximus, Hamstring group, Adductor group, namely Pectineus, Adductor brevis, Adductor longus, Adductor magnus, and Gracilis On side being stretched: Tensor fasciae latae and Gluteus minimus	Mainly on side being stretched: Abdominal group, especially Obliques, Latissimus dorsi, Quadratus lumborum, Erector spinae (lower aspect)	Rhomboids, Mid and Lower trapezius

STABILIZING MUSCLES

- Trunk: Abdominal group, Erector spinae, Quadratus lumborum
- Shoulder blades: Serratus anterior, Rhomboids, Lower trapezius
- Shoulders: Rotator cuff group, Deltoid

DIFFICULTY   **BEGINNER to ADVANCED**

WALKING ARM SWINGS

Dynamic/mobilization • Compound/multi-joint
Close chain • Bodyweight • Beginner to advanced

Given the shoulder's instability compared to the hip, warming up this joint is essential.

DESCRIPTION

While walking forwards, plantarflex the ankles and swing both arms in a forward direction in a circle for 10 to 20 arm swings. Then complete a further 10 to 20 arm swings in a backward direction while continuing to walk forwards, and plantarflex the ankles. Start slowly and increase the speed of movement as you warm up.

TRAINING TIPS

- Keep the torso upright.
- Ensure your arms brush your ears as you swing them past the head.
- Ensure you achieve full ankle plantarflexion as the arms pass directly overhead.

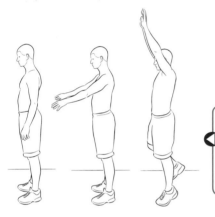

STARTING POSITION
- Stand with feet shoulder-width apart and torso upright, hands by your sides.

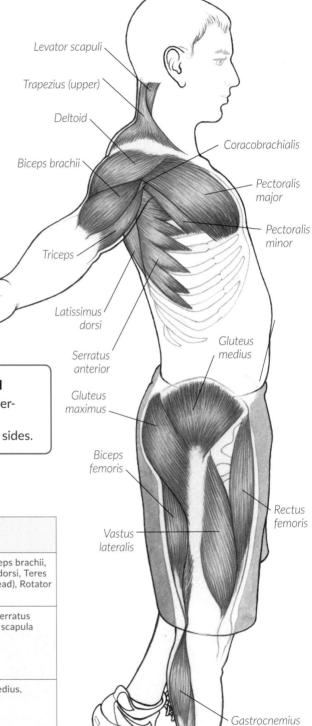

Levator scapuli
Trapezius (upper)
Deltoid
Biceps brachii
Triceps
Latissimus dorsi
Serratus anterior
Gluteus maximus
Biceps femoris
Vastus lateralis
Coracobrachialis
Pectoralis major
Pectoralis minor
Gluteus medius
Rectus femoris
Gastrocnemius
Soleus

ANALYSIS OF MOVEMENT	Joints	Joint movement	Mobilizing muscles
JOINT 1	Shoulder	Circumduction	Deltoid, Pectoralis major, Biceps brachii, Coracobrachialis, Latissimus dorsi, Teres major, Triceps brachii (long head), Rotator cuff
JOINT 2	Scapula	Upward rotation, abduction (protraction), downward rotation, adduction (retraction), elevation, depression	Trapezius, Pectoralis minor, Serratus anterior, Rhomboids, Levator scapula
JOINT 3	Hip	Back leg: extension, Forward leg: flexion	Gluteus maximus, Gluteus medius, Hamstring group
JOINT 4	Knee	Up: extension Down: flexion	Quadricep group
JOINT 5	Ankle	Up: plantarflexion Down: dorsiflexion	Gastrocnemius, Soleus, Tibialis posterior

KNEE-UPS

Dynamic/mobilization • Compound/multi-joint
Bodyweight • Beginner to advanced

This is an ideal warm-up for power and explosive work.

DESCRIPTION

Jog at a moderate speed, lifting the knees up in front of you until your knee hits your hand. Continue for 30–100 ft (10–30m).

TRAINING TIPS

- Keep the torso upright.
- Keep the foot contact with the ground as short as possible.

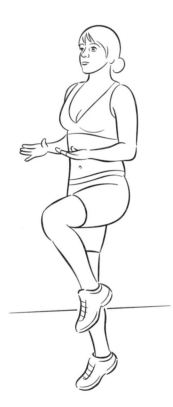

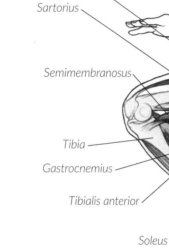

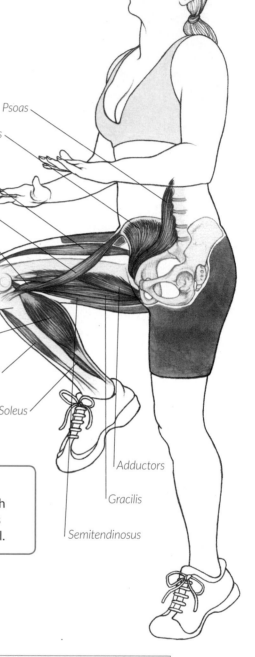

Psoas
Iliacus
Rectus femoris
Sartorius
Semimembranosus
Tibia
Gastrocnemius
Tibialis anterior
Soleus
Adductors
Gracilis
Semitendinosus

STARTING POSITION

- Stand with feet shoulder-width apart and torso upright, hands held in front of you at hip level.

ANALYSIS OF MOVEMENT	Joints	Joint movement	Mobilizing muscles
JOINT 1	Hip	Up: flexion Down: extension	Active leg: Iliopsoas, Tensor fascia latae, Rectus femoris
JOINT 2	Knee	Up: flexion Down: extension	Hamstring group, Gastrocnemius

HEEL KICKS

Dynamic/mobilization • Isolation/single joint
Bodyweight • Beginner to advanced

Heel kicks activate the hamstrings as well as the stabilization muscles around the hip area.

DESCRIPTION

Jog at a moderate speed flicking the legs back until the heels hit the hand. Continue for 30–100 ft (10–30m).

TRAINING TIPS

- Keep the torso upright.
- Keep the foot contact with the ground as short as possible.
- Lightly flick your hands with your heels.

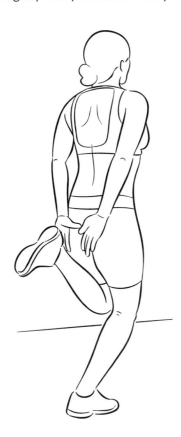

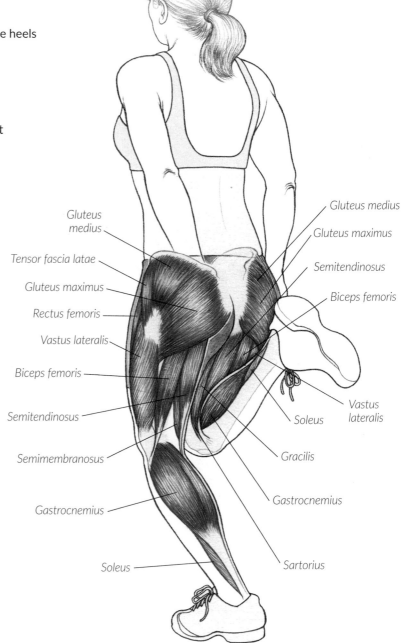

Gluteus medius

Tensor fascia latae

Gluteus maximus

Rectus femoris

Vastus lateralis

Biceps femoris

Semitendinosus

Semimembranosus

Gastrocnemius

Soleus

Gluteus medius

Gluteus maximus

Semitendinosus

Biceps femoris

Vastus lateralis

Soleus

Gracilis

Gastrocnemius

Sartorius

STARTING POSITION

- Stand with feet shoulder-width apart and torso upright, arms behind the body with the hands (palms facing backwards) on top of the gluteal muscles.

ANALYSIS OF MOVEMENT	Joints	Joint movement	Mobilizing muscles
JOINT 1	Knee	Up: flexion Down: extension	Hamstring group, Gastrocnemius

Abdominals, Stabilization, and Balance

ABDOMINAL MUSCLES

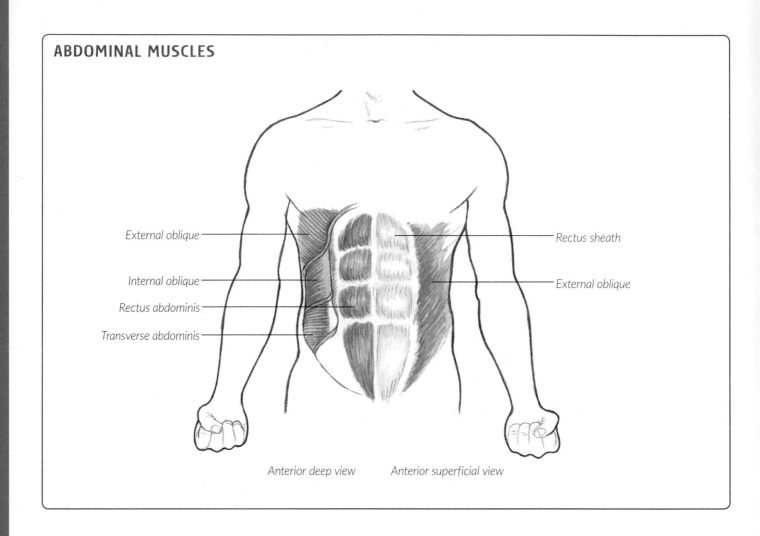

External oblique

Internal oblique

Rectus abdominis

Transverse abdominis

Rectus sheath

External oblique

Anterior deep view   Anterior superficial view

In functional fitness training (fitness training geared toward the requirements of day-to-day living), you want to train the muscles in the manner in which they were naturally intended to function.

Maintaining overall postural strength as well as relative strength-flexibility balance between opposing muscle groups (for example, the abdominals and lower back muscles) is key in functional fitness. Poor postural control affects the quality, safety, and effectiveness of your movements and exercises. It is likely to promote compensatory patterns, with the result that joints and muscles will not work in the manner they were intended to function. This increases the risk of injury and premature aging, as well as musculoskeletal problems that are typical of Western living.

Stabilizers are muscles whose prime purpose is to maintain the stability and alignment of the rest of the body, anchoring it effectively while other muscles perform the exercise or movement. For example, when doing barbell bicep curls, the rotator cuff muscles stabilize and align the shoulder area, the abdominal and lower back groups maintain the alignment of the spine, and the bicep muscles help lift the weight by flexing the elbow joints.

The abdominal group is one of several important stabilizers highlighted throughout this book. Other muscles that perform important stabilizing functions are discussed in more depth elsewhere in this book.

Major muscles of the lower anterior trunk

NAME	JOINTS CROSSED	ORIGIN	INSERTION	ACTION
Rectus abdominis	Anterior spine	Crest of the pubis	Xiphoid process and the cartilage of the 5th–7th ribs	Lumbar flexion (both sides); Lateral flexion to the right (right side); Lateral flexion to left (left side). Controls the posterior tilt of the pelvis (together with External obliques)
External obliques	Anterior spine	Lateral borders of the lower eight ribs	Four aspects: anterior side of the iliac crest; inguinal ligament; crest of the pubis; lower anterior fascia of the rectus abdominis	Lumbar flexion (both sides); Lumbar lateral flexion to the right and rotation to the left (right side); Lumbar lateral flexion to the left and rotation to right (left side). Controls the posterior tilt of the pelvis (together with the Rectus abdominis)
Internal obliques	Anterior spine	Three aspects: upper section of the inguinal ligament; anterior two-thirds of the crest of the ilium; the lumbar fascia	Costal cartilages of the 8th–10th ribs and linea alba (imagine a V-shape from hips to ribs)	Lumbar flexion (both sides); Lumbar lateral flexion and rotation to the right (right side); Lumbar lateral flexion and rotation to left (left side)
Transverse abdominis	Anterior spine	Four aspects: inguinal ligament; medial rim of iliac crest; medial surface of the lower six rib cartilages; the lumbar fascia	Three aspects: crest of the pubis; iliopectineal line; linea alba. It joins here with the transverse abdominis from the other side	The best type of contraction for this muscle is isometric, drawing the abdomen in toward the spine

Notes:

These muscles are listed in order from most superficial to deepest.

In rotating the trunk, the external and internal obliques combine (e.g., when the left elbow moves to the right knee, the left external obliques and the right internal obliques work together to rotate the trunk).

For other stabilizing muscles, see relevant sections.

DIFFICULTY   **BEGINNER to ADVANCED**

POSTURE PRIMER

Supine lying – Neutral spine with scapula release
Neutral spine – Stand and breathe
Core exercise • Whole body stabilization
• Beginner to advanced

Stabilizing muscles such as the abdominals help to maintain a posture balanced against the force of gravity. It is also important to learn how to stabilize the shoulder blades before doing strength work with the upper limbs to prevent the shoulders from hunching and rounding forwards, promoting neck pain. Relaxation breathing helps to relax the muscles and joints, and ensures a more stable postural base for exercise.

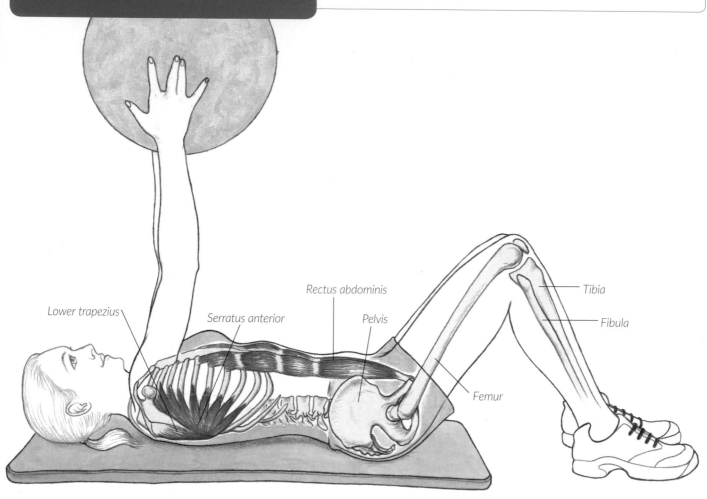

Lower trapezius · Serratus anterior · Rectus abdominis · Pelvis · Femur · Tibia · Fibula

SUPINE LYING – NEUTRAL SPINE WITH SCAPULA RELEASE

- Lie supine with a neutral spine and your legs either straight or bent.
- Hold a stability ball above your chest with your arms extended and your elbows soft.
- As you inhale, extend your arms toward the ceiling, gently rounding your shoulder blades forwards, but keeping your elbows soft.
- Relax your shoulder blades and let them settle into the mat.
- As your arms come down, gently depress them and wrap them forwards against the ribs, activating the Serratus anterior and Lower trapezius.
- You should be able to feel a little widening under your armpit at the side.
- Return and repeat.

SERRATUS ANTERIOR AND LOWER TRAPEZIUS

These two muscles stabilize the shoulder blades against the ribs. Learning to actively release and use them in your posture, as in this exercise, will counteract typical neck and shoulder tension.

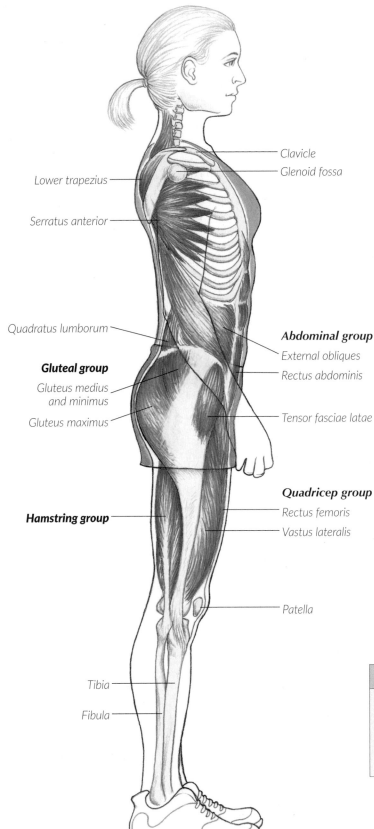

Lower trapezius

Serratus anterior

Quadratus lumborum

Gluteal group

Gluteus medius and minimus

Gluteus maximus

Hamstring group

Tibia

Fibula

Clavicle

Glenoid fossa

Abdominal group

External obliques

Rectus abdominis

Tensor fasciae latae

Quadricep group

Rectus femoris

Vastus lateralis

Patella

NEUTRAL SPINE – STAND AND BREATHE

- Keep your weight balanced through the middle of your feet.
- Breathe in deeply through your nose, feeling your ribcage open under your arms.
- Keep your heels down and imagine lifting your ankles and shin bones while you let out your breath naturally through your mouth.
- Soften your knees.
- Breathe in deeply again, this time "pulling" your quadriceps up from your knee. As you do so, rotate the upper thigh gently inwards. Feel it open space in your lower back as you let your breath out.
- Breathe in deeply again, gently lengthening your spine up from your pelvis. Gradually draw in your abdominal muscles, but let the coccyx down as you let out the breath.
- Breathe in deeply again, while lifting and opening your chest without sticking the lower border of your ribs forwards. Release your shoulder blades down and wrap forwards against your ribs as you let your breath out. You will feel the expansion under your arms.
- Relax your arms and shoulders.
- Breathing in again, gently lengthen your neck from the shoulders while balancing your head over your feet. Your eyes should look up slightly to the horizon as you let out your breath.

STABILIZING MUSCLES

- Abdominals, mainly the obliques and transverse
- Trunk: Quadratus lumborum, Erector spinae
- Shoulder blades: Serratus anterior, Rhomboids, Lower trapezius
- Legs and hips: Adductor group, Hamstring group, Rectus femoris, Gluteal group

ABDOMINAL STABILIZATION PROGRAM

Core exercise • Isolated • Stabilization focus on abdominals • Open chain • Bodyweight • Beginner to advanced

Adapted from the work of Shirley Sahrmann, a physical therapist who specializes in abdominal rehabilitation, this is a series of progressive exercises aimed at strengthening the stabilization strength of the abdominals and pelvic floor. The exercises are also ideal for restoring diastasis recti, a separation of the abdominal muscles that can occur during pregnancy. Most other abdominal work is unsuitable for pregnant and postpartum mothers, as it tends to create too much intra-abdominal pressure and back strain.

TRAINING TIPS

- Move to the next level when you can perform 20 repetitions on each side without discomfort or moving the back.
- Avoid momentum – use a slow, controlled movement.
- Avoid hunching your shoulders. Keep your chest open, head and spine neutral, and shoulder blades depressed.
- Avoid tensing the buttocks or forcing the lower back down into the mat. Concentrate on using the abdominals.

DESCRIPTION

It is important to master each level of this exercise before moving to the next.

STARTING POSITION

1. **Abdominal isolation -** Lie supine with your hips and knees bent, and your feet flat on the floor, hip-width apart. Keep your arms relaxed at your sides. Maintain a neutral spine, with abdominal stabilization engaged, mildly squeezing your navel into your spine without moving the spine. You should make sure you breathe easily as you squeeze, building up the time you hold the contraction.

ANALYSIS OF MOVEMENT	JOINT 1
Joints	Hip
Joint movement	Away from body – extension Return – flexion
Mobilizing muscles	Iliopsoas Rectus femoris

2. **Leg slide -** In the starting position and while maintaining a neutral spine and engaging abdominal stabilization, slowly slide one leg out until it is flat on the floor. Return, and relax the abdominals. Engage and repeat with the opposite leg.

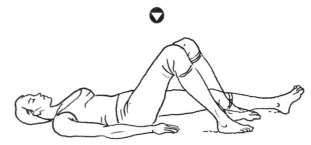

STABILIZING MUSCLES
• Abdominal group
• Neck: Sternocleidomastoid
• Shoulder blades: Serratus anterior, Rhomboids, Lower trapezius
• Hips: Iliopsoas, Rectus femoris

Note: *Most of the work in this exercise is performed by the stabilizing muscles.*

CAUTION: *If you have had a C-section, you can commence the exercise once the incision has healed. You should, however, obtain clearance from your obstetrician, gynecologist, or general practitioner before recommencing any exercise.*

3. **Knee raises -** From the starting position and while maintaining a neutral spine and engaging abdominal stabilization, raise one leg so that the knee is vertically above the hip and the lower leg is parallel with the ground. Return and repeat with the opposite leg.

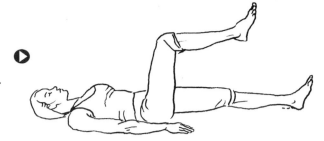

4. **Heel touch -** Now start from a similar position, but with your hips and knees bent at 90°, so that your knees are vertically above the hips and the lower leg is parallel with the ground. While maintaining a neutral spine and engaging abdominal stabilization, lower the heel of one leg to the ground. Maintain the 90° bend at the knee. Return and repeat with the opposite leg.

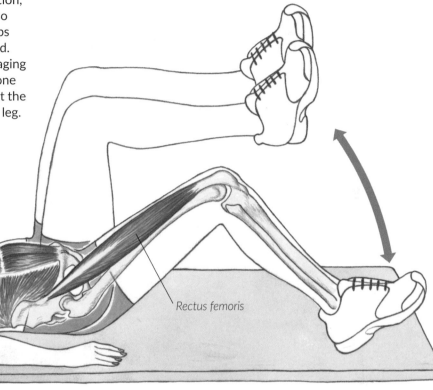

Sternocleidomastoid

Rectus abdominus

Rectus femoris

External obliques

Transverse abdominus

EXERCISE VARIATION AND PROGRESSION
Try using a stability ball for variety: for example, in Step 2 use a ball underfoot when you slide your leg out. To progress, you can add shoulder flexions: as the legs move away from the body the arms move in the opposite direction.

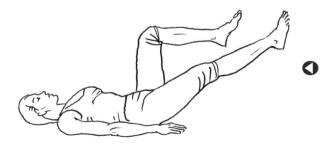

5. **Leg extensions -** Starting from the same position, with your hips and knees bent at 90° so that your knees are vertically above the hips and your lower leg is parallel with the ground, extend the leg straight out, keeping the foot 1–2 ft (30–60cm) off the ground. In the beginning you can extend the leg a shorter distance. As you master the exercise, extend further until the leg is fully extended.

TRANSVERSE ACTIVATION IN 4-POINT KNEELING

Whole-body stabilization • Isolation • Close chain • Bodyweight • Focus on abdominals • Beginner to advanced

This exercise helps to create awareness of and to strengthen the deepest abdominal, the Transverse abdominus, which helps to keep the abdomen flat and activates expulsion/expiration of the abdominal cavity.

DESCRIPTION

Inhale deeply. As you breathe out, squeeze the navel toward the spine, so that you see the abdominals moving upwards while the spine itself remains neutral. Relax and repeat.

TRAINING TIPS

- Use a slow, controlled, full range of movement.
- Avoid rounding or arching the mid and lower back. Keep the pelvis neutral and the spine aligned.
- Keep the chest open and shoulder blades depressed.
- As the transverse moves toward the spine, the waist just above the crest of the hip ("love handles") will seem to get smaller.

STARTING POSITION

- Kneel on all fours, with knees and hands directly under the hips and shoulders.
- Maintain a neutral spine.
- Keep the chest open. Aim to depress and widen the shoulder blades against the back, activating the Serratus anterior.

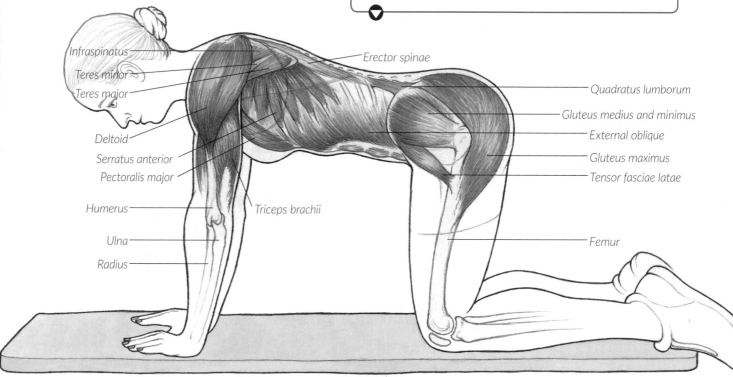

ANALYSIS OF MOVEMENT	JOINT 1
Joints	Trunk
Joint movement	None
Mobilizing muscles	Transverse abdominal

STABILIZING MUSCLES

- Trunk: Abdominals, mainly the Rectus, External and Internal oblique, Quadratus lumborum, Erector spinae, Adductor group, Gluteus medius and minimus
- Shoulder joint: Anterior deltoid, Pectoralis major, Rotator cuff muscles
- Shoulder blades: Serratus anterior, Rhomboids, Lower trapezius
- Arm: Triceps

DIFFICULTY | **INTERMEDIATE to ADVANCED**

FORWARD STABILITY BALL ROLL

Whole-body stabilization • Focus on abdominals, mid-back, shoulder stabilizers • Open chain • Bodyweight • Intermediate to advanced

The stability ball is an inflatable, heavy-duty, vinyl ball made to withstand repeated use. Introduced in 1909 as physical therapy for children with cerebral palsy, and later used for spinal injuries and back rehabilitation, it came into gym circles in the 1990s.

DESCRIPTION

Slowly roll forward maintaining a neutral spine, transverse activation and shoulder/scapula stabilization. Return and repeat.

TRAINING TIPS

- Avoid momentum. Use slow, controlled, full range of movement.
- The further forward you go, the longer the lever and the harder the exercise. Go only to the point where you can maintain effective stabilization, and build up from there.
- Avoid hunching or rounding the shoulders and dropping the hips or arching the back.
- Inhale on the forward phase.
- Start with fewer repetitions and build up.

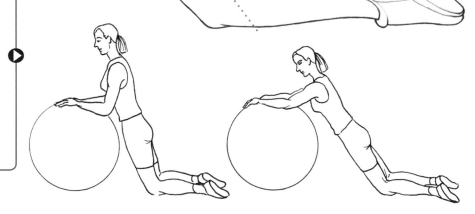

Supraspinatus
Infraspinatus
Teres minor
Teres major
Biceps brachii
Brachialis
Triceps brachii
Abdominal group
External oblique
Rectus abdominis
Superior anterior iliac crest
Serratus anterior
Latissimus dorsi
Quadratus lumborum
Iliac crest
Pelvis
Coccyx
Ischium
Ischial tuberosity

STARTING POSITION

- Start by kneeling, legs hip-width apart, in front of the stability ball.
- Place forearms on the ball and lean forward onto it.
- Keep your posture aligned and stabilized.
- Shoulders should be relaxed, the chest open, and the scapula depressed.

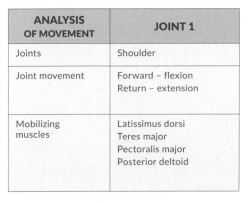

ANALYSIS OF MOVEMENT	JOINT 1
Joints	Shoulder
Joint movement	Forward – flexion Return – extension
Mobilizing muscles	Latissimus dorsi Teres major Pectoralis major Posterior deltoid

STABILIZING MUSCLES

- Abdominal group
- Trunk: Quadratus lumborum, Erector spinae, Adductor group, Gluteus medius and minimus
- Shoulder joint: Anterior Deltoid, Pectoralis major, Rotator cuff muscles
- Shoulder blades: Serratus anterior, Rhomboids, Lower trapezius
- Arm: Triceps brachii

PLANK POSE STABILIZATION

Whole-body stabilization • Focus on abdominals and mid-back stabilizers • Close chain • Bodyweight • Intermediate to advanced

Exercises such as the plank pose help to strengthen the stabilizing endurance of the abdominal muscles. This can, in turn, help to reduce the typical lower back pain associated with weak functional stability of the trunk muscles.

DESCRIPTION

The primary aim is to maintain stabilization and alignment for a period of time. Start with 10-second intervals and progress to 60 seconds.

TRAINING TIPS

- Avoid rounding or arching the back. Keep the pelvis neutral and the spine aligned.
- Avoid hanging on or hunching the shoulder blades. Keep the chest open and shoulder blades depressed.
- Do not hold your breath. Breathe in a relaxed manner.

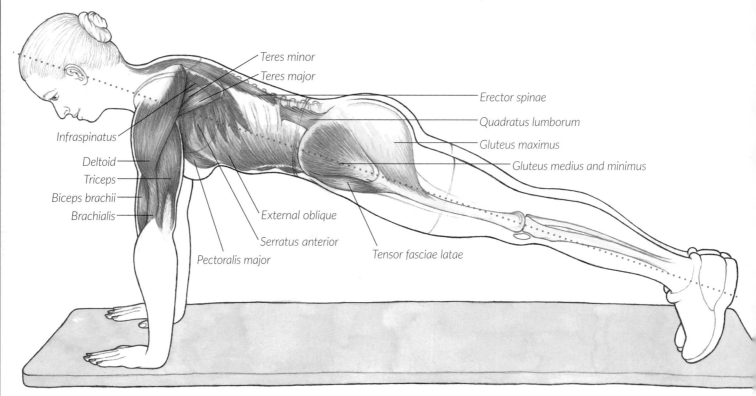

Teres minor
Teres major
Erector spinae
Quadratus lumborum
Gluteus maximus
Gluteus medius and minimus
Infraspinatus
Deltoid
Triceps
Biceps brachii
Brachialis
External oblique
Serratus anterior
Tensor fasciae latae
Pectoralis major

STARTING POSTITION

- Raise your body in the prone position, supported on hands and feet (hip-width apart).
- Extend your arms, slightly wider than shoulder-width, at the level of the upper chest.
- Maintain a neutral spine and engage abdominal stabilization, pulling your navel toward the spine.
- Keep your chest open. Aim to depress and widen the shoulder blades against the back, activating the Serratus anterior and lower Trapezius.

STABILIZING MUSCLES

- Abdominal group
- Trunk: Quadratus lumborum, Erector spinae, Adductor group, Gluteus medius and minimus
- Shoulder joint: Anterior deltoid, Pectoralis major, Rotator cuff muscles
- Shoulder blades: Serratus anterior, Rhomboids, Lower trapezius
- Arm: Biceps group, Triceps brachii

DIFFICULTY   **INTERMEDIATE to ADVANCED**

BODYWEIGHT LEANING SIDE ABDOMINAL

Whole-body stabilization • Abdominals, mid- and lower back, shoulder stabilizers • Close chain • Bodyweight • Intermediate to advanced

This exercise brings in the "sideways" stabilizers such as the Gluteus medius and minimus and the Adductors.

DESCRIPTION

The primary aim is to maintain the stabilization and alignment for a period of time. Start with 5-second intervals and progress to 30-second periods.

TRAINING TIPS

- Keep the shoulders relaxed, scapula depressed, and the abdominals stabilized.
- Avoid letting the top hip rotate forward.
- For an easier version, lower the body to lean on the right elbow.
- Keep the head and neck aligned with the spine.
- Swap over to train both left and right sides.

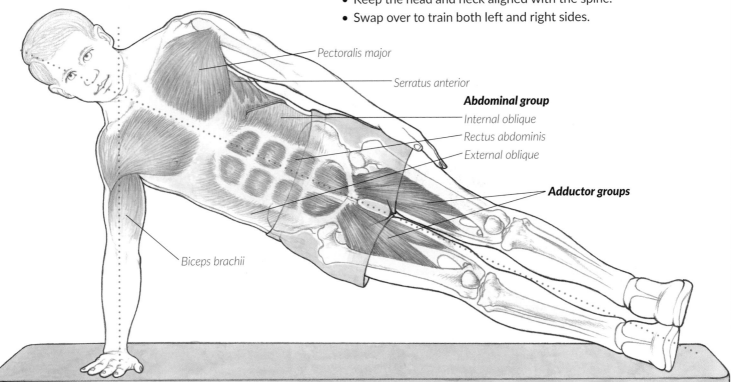

Pectoralis major
Serratus anterior
Abdominal group
Internal oblique
Rectus abdominis
External oblique
Adductor groups
Biceps brachii

STABILIZING MUSCLES

The main stabilizing emphasis is on the Abdominal group, particularly the Obliques and Transverse abdominus, and the Quadratus lumborum.

- Trunk: Erector spinae, Adductor group, Gluteus medius and minimus
- Shoulder joint: Deltoid, Rotator cuff muscles
- Shoulder blades: Serratus anterior, Rhomboids, Lower trapezius
- Arms: Bicep group, Triceps brachii

STARTING POSITION

- Sit on your right hip, knees bent.
- Keep the shoulder, hip, and knee in line.
- Lean on the right hand, underneath the right shoulder.
- Raise body at the hip, so that the midline of the body is straight.

DOUBLE LEG BRIDGE WITH SHOULDER FLEXION

Auxiliary exercise • Isolated/single joint • Push • Close chain • Bodyweight • Beginner to advanced

Bridge work was originally used in back rehabilitation and physical therapy. This adaptation is one of several core stability exercises that have made their way into gym routines.

DESCRIPTION

Slowly raise your trunk and lower back by extending your hips, keeping the arms relaxed. Pause, return, and repeat.

TRAINING TIPS

- Lead from the hips.
- Keep your knees hip-width apart.
- Keep your shoulders relaxed and your chest open.

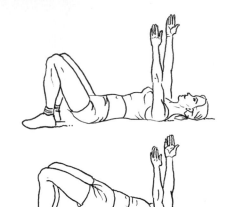

STARTING POSITION

- Lie supine with your knees bent and your feet flat.
- Raise your arms vertically toward the ceiling.
- Keep your shoulders relaxed and release your shoulder blades down.

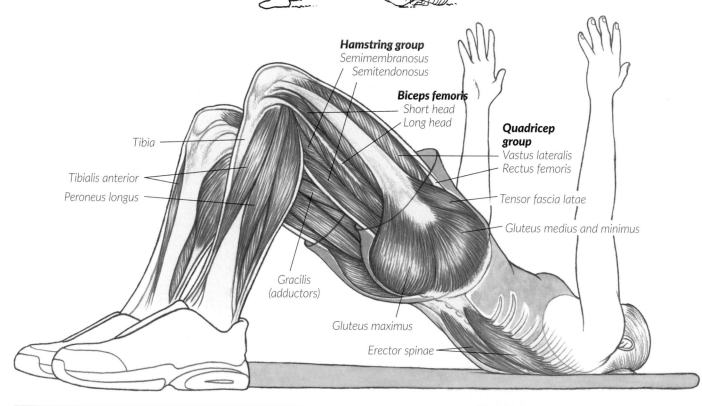

Hamstring group
Semimembranosus
Semitendonosus

Biceps femoris
Short head
Long head

Quadricep group
Vastus lateralis
Rectus femoris

Tensor fascia latae

Gluteus medius and minimus

Tibia

Tibialis anterior
Peroneus longus

Gracilis (adductors)

Gluteus maximus

Erector spinae

ANALYSIS OF MOVEMENT	JOINT 1
Joints	Hips
Joint movement	Up – extension Down – flexion
Mobilizing muscles	Gluteus maximus Hamstring group

STABILIZING MUSCLES

The main stabilizers are the Erector spinae, Abdominals, and Quadricep group. Additional stabilization:

- Shoulders: Rotator cuff group, Anterior deltoid
- Shoulder blades: Lower and Mid trapezius, Serratus anterior
- Trunk: Quadratus lumborum
- Hips: Gluteus medius and minimus, Deep lateral rotators, Adductor group

BALL BRIDGE

Whole-body stabilization • Push
• Close chain • Bodyweight
• Beginner to advanced

This exercise progresses bridging with the use of a stability ball under the lower legs.

DESCRIPTION

As you exhale, slowly raise your trunk and lower back by extending your hips, keeping your arm position relaxed. Pause, return, and repeat.

STARTING POSITION

- Lie supine with your knees bent, and your calf muscles on a stability ball.
- Keep your feet and knees hip-width apart.
- Keep your arms relaxed at your sides.
- Maintain a neutral spine, keep abdominal stabilization engaged, and mildly squeeze your navel to your spine without moving the spine.

TRAINING TIPS

- Work slowly and with control.
- Lead from the hips.
- Keep your knees hip-width apart.
- Keep your shoulders relaxed, your chest open, and the feeling of expansion under your arms.

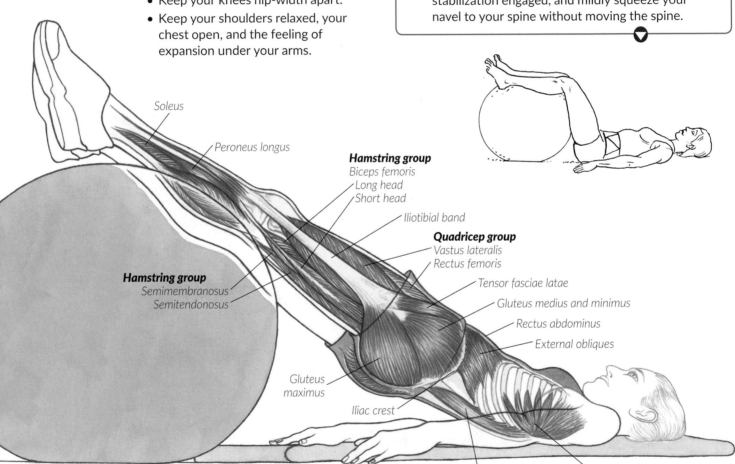

Soleus

Peroneus longus

Hamstring group
Biceps femoris
Long head
Short head

Iliotibial band

Quadricep group
Vastus lateralis
Rectus femoris

Tensor fasciae latae

Gluteus medius and minimus

Rectus abdominus

External obliques

Hamstring group
Semimembranosus
Semitendonosus

Gluteus maximus

Iliac crest

Erector spinae

Serratus anterior

ANALYSIS OF MOVEMENT	JOINT 1
Joints	Hips
Joint movement	Up – extension Down – flexion
Mobilizing muscles	Gluteus maximus Hamstring group

STABILIZING MUSCLES

The main stabilizers are the Erector spinae, Abdominals, and Quadricep group. Additional stabilization:

- Shoulder blades: Lower and Mid trapezius, Serratus anterior
- Trunk: Quadratus lumborum
- Hips: Gluteus medius and minimus, Deep lateral rotators, Adductor group

BODYWEIGHT CRUNCHES

Auxiliary exercise • Isolated • Pull
• Open chain • Bodyweight
• Beginner to advanced

Crunch exercises primarily work the abdominals as a mobilizer. The many variations are useful in any ab training program. (Note: Tight back-extensor muscles, such as the Erector spinae, will inhibit possible peak contraction and range of motion in the crunch.)

TRAINING TIPS

- Avoid momentum. Use a slow, controlled full range of movement.
- Avoid forcing the neck or chin to lift the body. Keep the chin tucked in slightly and neutral with the cervical spine as you curl up.
- Avoid pulling the trunk up with the hands. Rather, activate and isolate the abdominals.
- Avoid hunching the shoulders. Keep the chest open and the shoulder blades depressed.
- Exhale on the up phase.

DESCRIPTION

Slowly curl the upper body upwards by flexing the trunk. The scapula should lift off the mat, but the lower back remains on it, stable and neutral. Pause, return, and repeat. (Folding the arms across the chest makes the exercise easier, but will reduce neck support.)

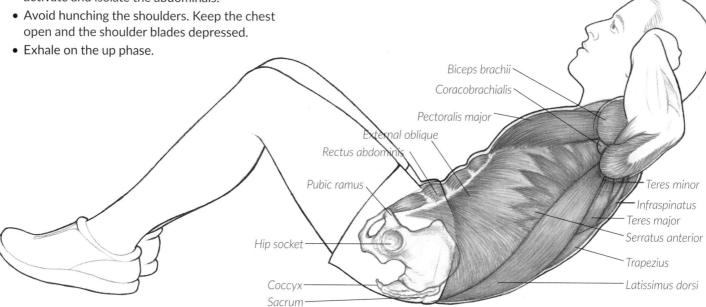

Biceps brachii
Coracobrachialis
Pectoralis major
External oblique
Rectus abdominis
Pubic ramus
Hip socket
Coccyx
Sacrum
Teres minor
Infraspinatus
Teres major
Serratus anterior
Trapezius
Latissimus dorsi

STARTING POSITION

- Lie supine with knees bent and feet flat.
- Clasp hands behind the head.
- Maintain neutral alignment in the cervical spine.
- Keep abdominal stabilization active.

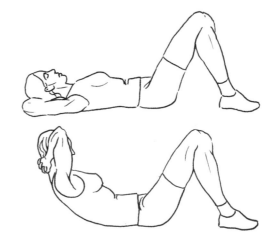

ANALYSIS OF MOVEMENT	JOINT 1
Joints	Spine
Joint movement	Up – flexion Down – extension
Mobilizing muscles	Rectus abdominals and obliques

STABILIZING MUSCLES	The Abdominal group Neck: Sternocleidomastoid Shoulder blades: Serratus anterior, Rhomboids, and Lower trapezius

DIFFICULTY   **INTERMEDIATE to ADVANCED**

BODYWEIGHT SIT-UPS

Core exercise • Compound/multi-joint
• Pull • Open chain • Bodyweight
• Intermediate to advanced

Sit-ups have gained a bad reputation, mainly because of poor technique and instruction. Yet, done correctly, this is an effective and advanced compound exercise. The focus should be on quality of movement, not high velocity or frequent repetitions.

TRAINING TIPS

- Avoid momentum. Use a slow, controlled, full range of movement.
- Avoid forcing the neck or chin forward as you lift the body. Keep the chin tucked in slightly and neutral with the cervical spine as you curl up.
- Avoid pulling the trunk up with the hands. Rather, activate and isolate the abdominals.
- Avoid hunching the shoulders. Keep the chest open and shoulder blades depressed.
- Exhale on the up phase.
- Do fewer repetitions without any support, rather than more repetitions with the feet being held. With the feet held and increased velocity, momentum will be generated, leveraged against the lower back. This puts the lower back at risk.

DESCRIPTION

Slowly curl the upper body by flexing the trunk. Complete the trunk flexion, bringing the upper body toward the knees. Pause, return slowly, and repeat.

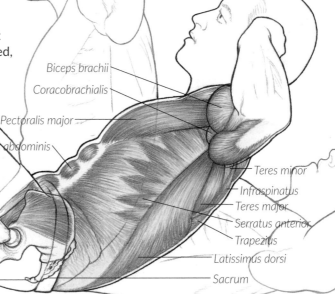

Biceps brachii
Coracobrachialis
Pectoralis major
Rectus abdominis
Teres minor
Infraspinatus
Teres major
Serratus anterior
Trapezius
Latissimus dorsi
Coccyx
Sacrum

STARTING POSITION

- Lie supine with knees bent and feet flat.
- Keep your hands unclasped behind your head.
- Maintain neutral alignment in the cervical spine.
- Keep the abdominal stabilization active.

ANALYSIS OF MOVEMENT	PHASE 1 FIRST ±30° SAME AS CRUNCH RANGE OF MOVEMENT	PHASE 2 REMAINDER OF MOVEMENT TO RAISE LOWER BACK
Joints	Spine	Hip
Joint movement	Up – flexion Down – extension	Up – flexion Down – extension
Mobilizing muscles	Rectus abdominals and obliques	Iliopsoas, Rectus femoris
Stabilizing muscles	Neck: Sternocleidomastoid Shoulder blades: Serratus anterior, Rhomboids, and Lower trapezius	Neck: Rectus abdominals and obliques, Sternocleidomastoid Shoulder blades: Serratus anterior, Rhomboids, and Lower trapezius

DIFFICULTY ADVANCED

HANGING LEG RAISES

Whole-body stabilization • Focus on abdominals, mid- and lower back, and shoulder stabilizers • Close chain • Bodyweight • Advanced

This effective, but advanced, exercise is not suitable for anyone with poor core stabilization ability, or shoulder or back problems.

DESCRIPTION

Raise knees to hip height, maintaining a stabilized trunk. Return and repeat.

TRAINING TIPS

- Avoid momentum. Use controlled movements.
- Avoid collapsing the scapula so that the shoulders look hunched. Raise the body by depressing the scapula through the action of the lower Trapezius and Serratus anterior.
- Keep the chest open.

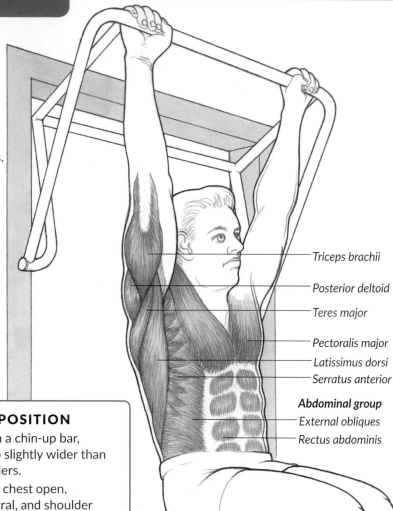

- Triceps brachii
- Posterior deltoid
- Teres major
- Pectoralis major
- Latissimus dorsi
- Serratus anterior

Abdominal group
- External obliques
- Rectus abdominis

STARTING POSITION

- Hang from a chin-up bar, with a grip slightly wider than the shoulders.
- Keep your chest open, spine neutral, and shoulder blades depressed.
- Legs should dangle, but abdominals stabilize the pelvis.

ANALYSIS OF MOVEMENT	JOINT 1
Joints	Hip
Joint movement	Up – flexion Down – extension
Mobilizing muscles	Iliopsoas Rectus femoris

STABILIZING MUSCLES

- Abdominal group
- Shoulder blades: Serratus anterior, Rhomboids, Lower trapezius
- Shoulders: Latissimus dorsi, Rotator cuff group

DIFFICULTY | **INTERMEDIATE to ADVANCED**

STANDING SQUAT (BOSU BALANCE TRAINER)

Whole-body stabilization and balance focus
• Close chain • Bodyweight • Intermediate to advanced

BOSU is an acronym for "Both-Sides-Up." This balance trainer is like a stability ball cut in half, with a platform on the bottom. It can be used ball-side up to challenge lower body balance and stability, or platform-side up to target upper body strength.

DESCRIPTION

Standing on the BOSU trainer, flex your knees and squat, as though you're sitting back in a chair. Extend your arms to the front to help maintain your balance. Return to a standing position and repeat.

TRAINING TIPS

- If pelvic stabilization cannot be maintained, lower less than 90° at the knees. Start with as little as 45° flexion.

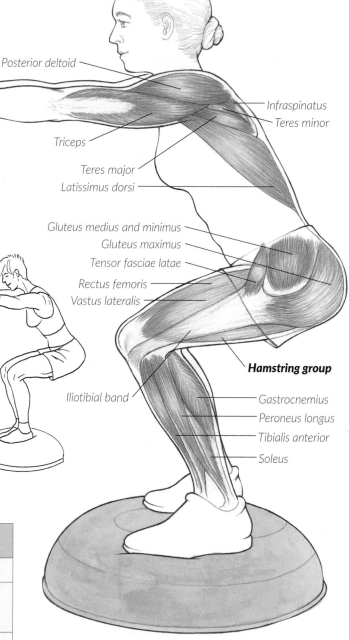

Posterior deltoid
Infraspinatus
Teres minor
Triceps
Teres major
Latissimus dorsi
Gluteus medius and minimus
Gluteus maximus
Tensor fasciae latae
Rectus femoris
Vastus lateralis
Hamstring group
Iliotibial band
Gastrocnemius
Peroneus longus
Tibialis anterior
Soleus

STARTING POSITION

- Stand on the BOSU with your feet placed slightly forward of the center.
- Keep knees soft, and your posture aligned and stabilized.

STABILIZING MUSCLES

- Trunk: Abdominal group, Erector spinae, Quadratus lumborum
- Hips: Gluteus medius and minimus, deep external rotators, Adductor group
- Ankle stabilizers

ANALYSIS OF MOVEMENT	JOINT 1	JOINT 2
Joints	Knee	Hip
Joint movement	Down – flexion Up – extension	Down – flexion Up – extension
Mobilizing muscles	Quadricep group	Hamstring group Gluteus maximus

Compound and Power Exercises

Powerlifting is a strength sport consisting of three lifts, namely, the squat, bench press, and dead lift. Weightlifting, also called Olympic-style weightlifting, or Olympic weightlifting, is an athletic sport on the modern Olympic program featuring two competitions: the snatch and the clean and jerk. In powerlifting and Olympic weightlifting, aesthetics is secondary to the objective of lifting the most weight. CrossFit uses a fair amount of high-repetition Olympic lifting, whereas bodybuilding uses a combination of compound and isolation exercises to build the muscle mass.

The move away from gym machine training and toward functional, compound training has seen an increase in interest in using traditional powerlifting and weightlifting exercises, as well as the inclusion of chin-ups, overhead press, gymnastics, kettlebell, medicine ball, and other strongman exercises.

Power is a combination of the strength and speed domains. A powerful or explosive movement is one that involves relatively fast and forceful actions. Weights lifted can be measured in terms of percentage of 1 repetition max (1RM): the maximum weight you can lift properly, in each exercise, once and only once.

In power training, it is generally agreed that lower weights (about 30% of 1RM) and higher velocity will improve the speed, as well as plyometric explosive aspects, while workloads greater than 85% of 1RM will improve the maximal strength component. Between 30%–70% will divide improvements between both components and is considered the "power zone" (see the graph here).

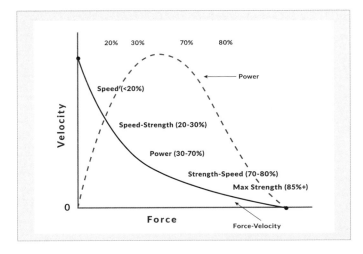

It takes time to adapt to power exercise. Therefore, it is generally recommended for beginners to work with lower weights (about 30%) and to focus on good form.

When you add an external load to an exercise, you cannot do the movement at the same velocity as when the movement is non-weighted. The more weight you add to a movement, the greater the variance in biomechanics you will likely see, especially if velocity is high. This is one reason why people might become injured when lifting very heavy loads in the weight room, as they alter their body mechanics to compensate for weaker segments in the body.

Each strength sport and exercise type has its own priority and training goal. So although we can adjust which variables of speed, strength, and endurance predominate, the principle of SAID will always apply. If the emphasis is on speed, then strength and endurance will diminish, as the anaerobic energy systems fade quickly. Likewise, if maximal strength is the focus, velocity will be slower, as one must move a heavier weight. Endurance will also be compromised as fatigue sets in early. Finally, if endurance is the focus, weight and speed must drop.

So, of the three variables (speed, strength, and endurance), we can place emphasis on one or two, but not all three at the same time (see the figure below).

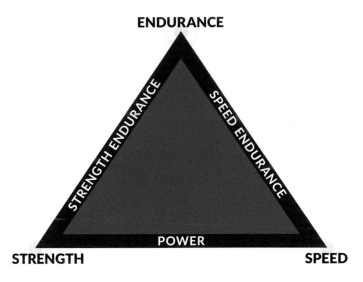

Caution: Power exercises are explosive, fluid, and continuous in nature and incorporate momentum. They are more advanced exercises. They can lead to severe injury if not performed correctly or if you are not suitably conditioned for them. For these reasons, you should not attempt to do the exercises in this section without proper instruction and initial supervision. These exercises are not suitable for beginners or for those not yet fit enough, and should not be attempted if you have any neck, back, knee, or other significant injuries.

DIFFICULTY   **INTERMEDIATE to ADVANCED**

BENT LEG GOOD MORNING

- *Auxiliary exercise* • *Isolated/single joint* • *Pull*
- *Closed chain* • *Barbell*
- *Intermediate to advanced*

This exercise, which derives its name from its rising movement, takes one back to the classic bodybuilding era of the 1950s and 1960s, before back extension machines were built, yet its application is timeless.

DESCRIPTION

Lower the trunk by flexing at the hips until the trunk is parallel with the floor. Bend the knees slightly during the descent. Return to the starting position and repeat.

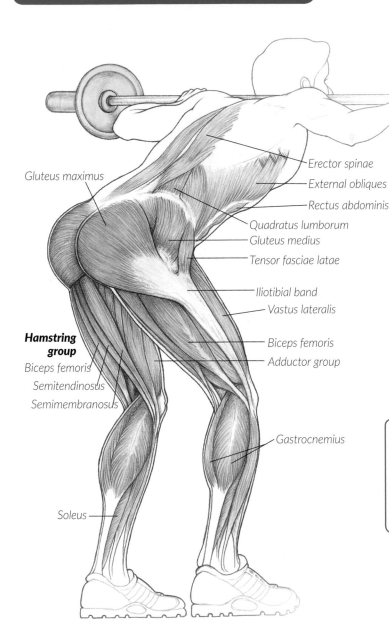

- Gluteus maximus
- Erector spinae
- External obliques
- Rectus abdominis
- Quadratus lumborum
- Gluteus medius
- Tensor fasciae latae
- Iliotibial band
- Vastus lateralis
- **Hamstring group**
- Biceps femoris
- Semitendinosus
- Semimembranosus
- Biceps femoris
- Adductor group
- Gastrocnemius
- Soleus

TRAINING TIPS

- Get a proper demonstration and instructions before doing this exercise.
- Good form is more important than the weight lifted. Start with a very light weight and use a smaller range of motion until you adapt.
- Maintain posture stabilization.
- Avoid rounding the back; keep it aligned.
- The less the hamstring flexibility, the more the knees will need to be bent in order to keep the back straight and maintain lumbar curvature.
- Inhale on the downward phase; exhale on the upward movement.

STARTING POSITION

- Stand with your feet shoulder-width apart; keep your knees soft.
- Place the barbell across the back of your shoulders (Posterior deltoid/Upper trapezius).

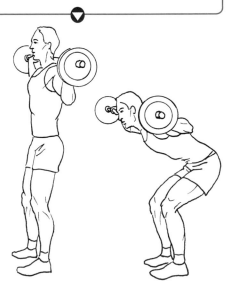

ANALYSIS OF MOVEMENT	JOINT 1
Joints	Hips
Joint movement	Down – flexion Up – extension
Mobilizing muscles	Gluteus maximus Hamstring group

STABILIZING MUSCLES

The main stabilizers are the Erector spinae and Quadricep group. Additional stabilization:

- Shoulder blades: Lower and Mid trapezius, Levator scapula, Rhomboids, Serratus anterior
- Abdominal group
- Hips: Gluteus medius and minimus, Deep lateral rotators, Adductor group, Quadratus lumborum
- Lower leg: Ankle stabilizers, Tibialis anterior, Gastrocnemius

BODYWEIGHT/AIR SQUAT

Core exercise • Compound/multi-joint • Close chain • Bodyweight • Beginner to intermediate

The squat is one of the most basic core movements. This page focuses on the mechanical basics of posture and alignment. It is essential these are correct before proceeding to all leg, compound, and power exercises.

DESCRIPTION

BASIC SQUAT:

Slowly lower the body, moving the hips back as if sitting into a chair. Beginners should lower to approximately 90° of knee flexion: stop before the upper leg becomes parallel with the floor. Return and repeat.

DEEP KNEE/AIR SQUAT:

You can go into a deep knee squat, provided you have no joint or injury limitations, and you are able to maintain proper form. Return and repeat.

SQUATTING PRIMER

The squat is one of the most important core exercises in all resistance training modalities. Known by many names, the bodyweight version (i.e., without added weights) is the foundation for all progressions into the back squat, front squat, and overhead squat, as well as the Olympic lifts and a range of other power exercises. The simple bodyweight squat was featured in the previous edition of this book. This edition now also examines the air squat, CrossFit's term for a deep knee bodyweight squat.

Deep Knee Bends and Risk

Although common exercise guidelines stress limiting deep knee bends, due to the greater injury risk, these are written with the broad and general population in mind, for many of whom deep knee bends do pose an increased risk. That said, in the absence of contraindications and real limitations, and with quality, educated instruction and proper progression, the deep knee squat can be a safe and effective progression in your training program. A good instructor will take into account the level of fitness of the individual, their weight, and their injury history before proceeding with a deep knee squat.

SIGNS	PROBLEM	CORRECTION
Lifting the heels off the ground	Poor ankle flexibility, limited dorsiflexion	• Perform proper warm-up and stretching, including ankle mobilizations, dynamic, and PNF stretching • Improve the functional flexibility of the calf muscles • Use foam roller on calves • Consider professional myofascial release and manual therapy
Rounding of the lumbar curve (Kyphosis)	Tends to be most common problem. Tight hamstrings and hip flexors. Poor pelvic control	• Lift the chest or raise the arms forward during descent into the squat • Learn to brace and maintain lumbar curvature • Perform proper warm-up and stretching, including ankle mobilizations, dynamic, and PNF stretching • Improve the functional flexibility of the hamstring muscles • Consider professional myofascial release and manual therapy
Dropping of the head, rounding forward of the chest and shoulders	Loss of neutral cervical and thoracic spine. Weakness of upper back stabilizers (i.e., Lower traps, Serratus anterior). Tightness of chest muscles	• Angle the head and eyes to look slightly above horizon throughout the movement
Knees rolling inward of feet as you squat. Specifically, the medial knee cap moves inward of the big toe as you squat	Usually the result of a lack of gluteal muscle and abductor activation, to control lateral movement of the knee	• Use verbal cues to "push the knees out" or place greater emphasis on the lateral sole of the foot • Use a ball between the knees to prevent collapsing of the knees inward • Use band around knees to heighten external rotation of hip • Start with a wider stance • In all leg presses and squats, keep the feet flat and press through the center of the foot to increase the activation of the Gluteus maximus muscle
In women, specifically, medial rotation of the knees in squatting. Knees roll inward, i.e., knock-kneed as woman squats	Predisposed by women having wider pelvis and more oblique carriage angle from hip to knee	• Place your feet wider than shoulder-width in the starting position
Not going deep enough, in the absence of contraindications	Lack of basic functional hamstring, glutes, and quadricep strength. Lack of functional postural strength and body awareness	• Encourage deeper squats with a box and later a medicine ball behind • Perform Quadricep stretching

STARTING POSITION

- Stand, feet shoulder distance apart, with knees soft.
- Keep posture aligned, with a neutral spine.
- Cross arms in front of body.

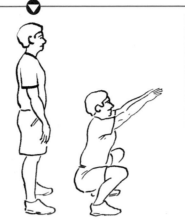

In the absence of contraindications to squatting and deep knee squats, the two most important areas to address are joint flexibility and neuromuscular control. Deficiencies in these areas are the most common faults that must be addressed before progressing to more advanced and weighted compound leg exercises. This primer will help you ensure that the basic foundation is solid and correct before you proceed to scaled-up and more complex whole body and power exercises.

ANALYSIS OF MOVEMENT	JOINT 1	JOINT 2
Joints	Hip	Knee
Joint movement	Down – flexion Up – extension	Down – flexion Up – extension
Mobilizing muscles	Gluteus maximus Hamstring group	Quadricep group

Technical note: *The deep knee squat increases the range of motion of the hip, knee, and ankle joints and therefore the work of the muscles that move those joints. It also increases the requirements of flexibility, neuromuscular control, and postural stabilization.*

Essential Points

1. **Movement quality, i.e., good form, and good synchronized coordination of the movement must precede the basic foundation of strength development, which in turn should precede speed/power development.**

2. **Learn to brace and maintain the lumbar spine.**

3. **Angle the head and eyes to look slightly above the horizon throughout the movement.**

4. **Learn to stand with soft knees: knees not hyperextended backward.**

5. **Keep weight distributed between the three points of the soles of the feet.**

6. **Don't let the knees collapse inward, or force the weight through the big toe and forefoot. Keep your feet flat, and avoid lifting the heels.**

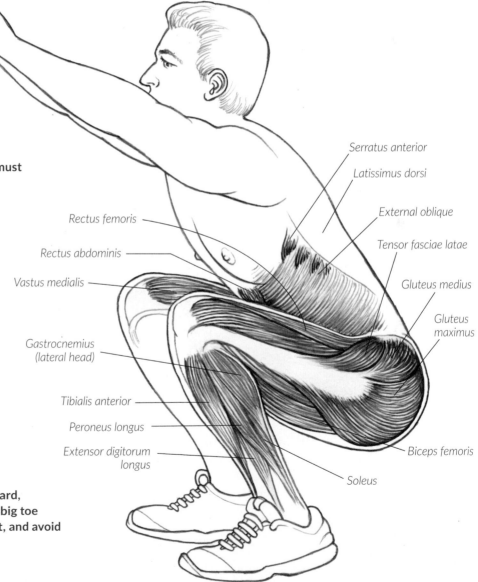

Rectus femoris

Rectus abdominis

Vastus medialis

Gastrocnemius (lateral head)

Tibialis anterior

Peroneus longus

Extensor digitorum longus

Serratus anterior

Latissimus dorsi

External oblique

Tensor fasciae latae

Gluteus medius

Gluteus maximus

Biceps femoris

Soleus

BACK SQUAT

Core exercise • Compound/multi-joint
• Push • Closed chain • Barbell
• Intermediate to advanced

The back squat has broad value and application in training, from heavy-duty bodybuilding to functional training and back rehabilitation. The stresses placed on the joints and muscles during closed chain movements are more functional and offer more natural stresses on the body when compared with open chain exercises.

DESCRIPTION

Slowly lower the body, moving the hips back as if sitting on a chair. Lower to approximately 90° of knee flexion: stop before the upper leg becomes parallel with the floor. Return and repeat.

TRAINING TIPS

- Establish good form before increasing weight.
- Avoid momentum; use slow, controlled movements.
- Keep posture aligned and the spine neutral.
- Keep your chest open, and avoid rounding the shoulders.
- Keep the knees from passing over the vertical line of the toes.
- Keep your weight directly over the heel to mid-foot. Avoid lifting the heels.
- If lumbar curvature cannot be maintained, lower to less than 90°. Start with as little as 45° movement at knee.
- Inhaling on the downward phase helps to increase intra-abdominal pressure, which keeps the shoulders open, and prevents spinal flexion. Exhale on the upward movement.

STARTING POSITION

- Take the bar off the squat rack and move back into a safe space for squatting.
- Stand, with feet shoulder-width apart, with soft knees.
- Hold the bar wider than the shoulders, as is comfortable.

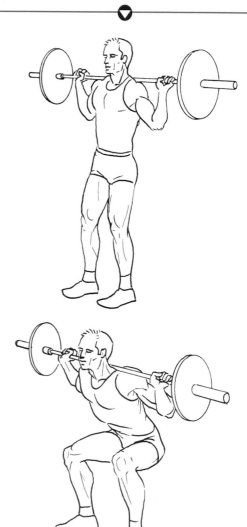

ANALYSIS OF MOVEMENT	JOINT 1	JOINT 2
Joints	Hip	Knee
Joint movement	Down – flexion Up – extension	Down – flexion Up – extension
Mobilizing muscles	Gluteus maximus Hamstring group	Quadricep group

STABILIZING MUSCLES

- Trunk: Abdominal group, Erector spinae, Quadratus lumborum
- Hips: Gluteus medius and minimus, Deep lateral rotators, Adductor group
- Lower leg: Ankle stabilizers, Gastrocnemius

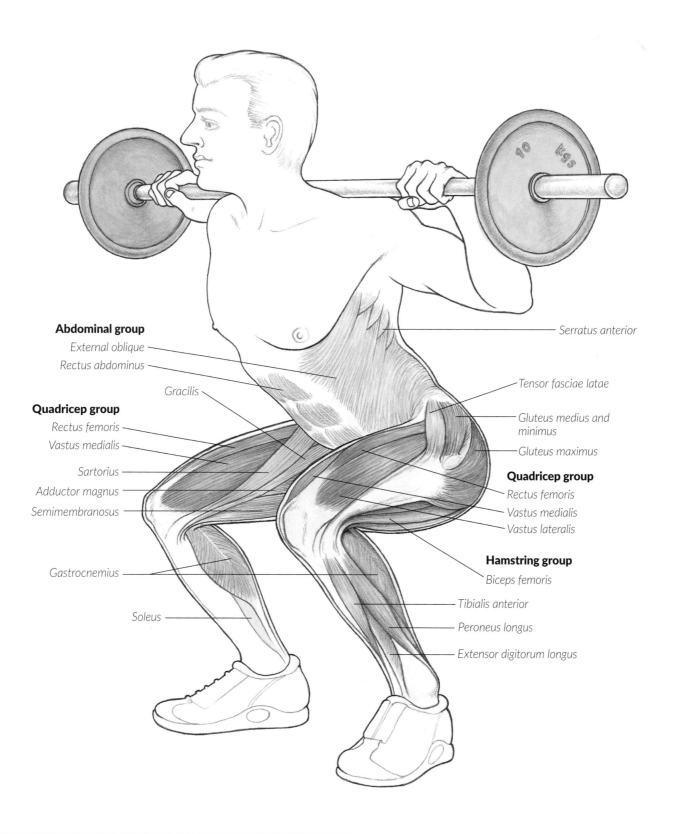

Abdominal group
External oblique
Rectus abdominus

Gracilis

Quadricep group
Rectus femoris
Vastus medialis

Sartorius

Adductor magnus

Semimembranosus

Gastrocnemius

Soleus

Serratus anterior

Tensor fasciae latae

Gluteus medius and minimus

Gluteus maximus

Quadricep group
Rectus femoris
Vastus medialis
Vastus lateralis

Hamstring group
Biceps femoris

Tibialis anterior

Peroneus longus

Extensor digitorum longus

CAUTION: If you experience any form of knee pain, do not proceed with this exercise. Beginners should get advice on what weight to start with.

FRONT SQUAT

*Core exercise • Compound/multi-joint •
Push • Close chain • Barbell • Intermediate
to advanced*

In recent years, the front squat has gained in popularity, mainly through CrossFit and functional training programming. Though it requires greater flexibility and offers greater challenge to lumbar stabilization, it allows a deeper squat while maintaining the center of gravity, places greater emphasis on the Quadriceps than the back squat, and better prepares one for the more complex Olympic lifts.

DESCRIPTION

Slowly lower the body, moving the hips back as if sitting into a chair. Beginners should lower to approximately 90° of knee flexion: stop before the upper leg becomes parallel with the floor. Advanced practitioners can go into a deep knee squat, provided you have no joint or injury limitations and that you are able to maintain proper form. Return and repeat.

TRAINING TIPS

- Perfect the air squat technique as foundation (see page 58).
- Achieve good form before increasing weight. Avoid momentum. Use controlled movement.
- Keep the posture aligned and the spine neutral. Brace and maintain the arch of the lumbar spine. Keep chest open, avoiding rounding the shoulders.
- Keep the knees from passing over the vertical line of the toes and keep your weight directly over the mid foot. Avoid lifting the heels.
- If lumbar curvature cannot be maintained, do not deep knee bend. Go back to the squatting primer. Start with as little as 45° movement at knee.
- Do not progress if you have knee pain in this exercise/limit deep knee bends.
- Inhalation on the downward phase helps to increase intra-abdominal pressure.
- The flexibility of the wrists and elbows required for the cradle grip makes it nearly impossible to hold a perfect front squat position for many new athletes. Pre-stretching the wrist helps.

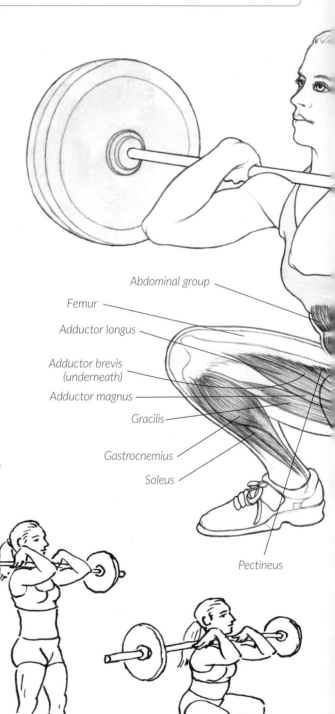

Abdominal group

Femur

Adductor longus

Adductor brevis (underneath)

Adductor magnus

Gracilis

Gastrocnemius

Soleus

Pectineus

STARTING POSITION

- Take the bar off the squat rack safely and move back into a safe space for squatting.
- Stand with your feet shoulder distance apart.
- The bar rests on chest and shoulders, held in place by loose cradle grip, with elbows high and forward.
- Keep posture aligned, with a neutral spine, knees soft.

STABILIZING MUSCLES

- Abdominal group, Erector spinae, and Quadratus lumborum at the trunk
- Gluteus medius and minimus, Deep lateral rotators, and the Adductor group at the hips
- Ankle stabilizers and Gastrocnemius in the lower leg

HOW TO LEARN TO SQUAT WITH A BAR

Start freestanding squats (see the squatting primer on page 58) with a broomstick on the shoulders and a chair/box/ball behind you as you squat. The broomstick gives you a sense of carrying the weight on your shoulders, and the chair gets you to bring the hips back to the right depth, while offering some security.

Then learn how to take an unweighted bar from the squat rack. On the rack, the bar should be at upper chest height, so that at the pickup, your knees are bent. Dip your upper body underneath the bar for a back squat.

Position the bar on the "meat" of your shoulders on the upper Trapezius. Commonly, women experience more discomfort with the bar placement across the upper Trapezius, having less soft tissue and a smaller area on which to place the bar. One recommendation is to emphasize opening the shoulders and chest. This will relax the tissues of the upper Trapezius, providing a better cushion for the bar. In some gyms, padded bar rolls are also available.

Inhale, keep your eyes looking slightly above the horizon, and then pick up the bar by standing up into the weight. When ready, walk back into the start position.

Follow the reverse procedure for taking the bar off.

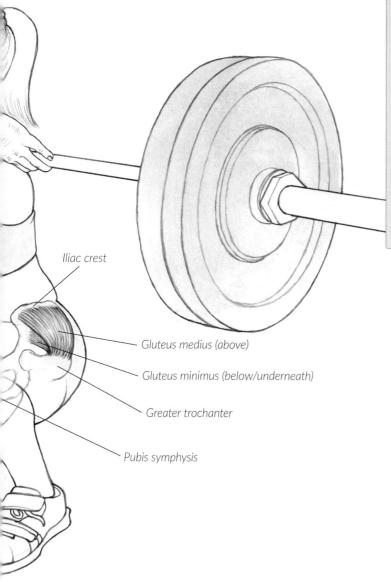

Iliac crest

Gluteus medius (above)

Gluteus minimus (below/underneath)

Greater trochanter

Pubis symphysis

DUMBBELL FRONT SQUAT

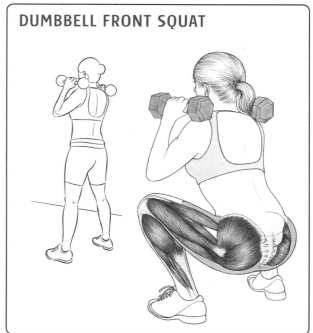

ANALYSIS OF MOVEMENT	JOINT 1	JOINT 2
Joints	Hip	Knee
Joint movement	Down – flexion Up – extension	Down - flexion Up - extension
Mobilizing muscles	Gluteus maximus Hamstring group	Quadricep group

DIFFICULTY   ADVANCED

OVERHEAD SQUAT

Core exercise • Compound/multi-joint • Push •
Close chain • Barbell • Advanced

By raising the center of mass with the additional requirement of stabilization of an overhead load, the overhead squat is arguably one of the most challenging exercises in stabilization. It easily highlights flaws in squat form and posture.

DESCRIPTION

Slowly lower the body, moving the hips back as if sitting into a chair. Beginners should lower to approximately 90° of knee flexion: stop before the upper leg becomes parallel with the floor. Advanced practitioners can go into a deep knee squat, provided no joint or injury limitations, and you are able to maintain proper form. Return and repeat.

TRAINING TIPS

- Perfect the bodyweight/air squat technique as a foundation for this exercise.
- Start this exercise using a broomstick and perfect good form before increasing weight. In particular, always maintain the bar directly overhead—do not let it move forward.
- Avoid momentum. Use slow, controlled movement.
- Keep the posture aligned and the spine neutral. Brace and maintain the arch of the lumbar spine.
- Keep the chest open and avoid rounding the shoulders.
- Keep the knees from passing over the vertical line of the toes.
- Keep your weight directly over the heel to mid-foot. Avoid lifting the heels.
- Don't drop the head; maintain eye level just above the horizon with a neutral cervical spine.
- If lumbar curvature cannot be maintained, do not use a deep knee bend. Go back to the squatting primer.
- Start with as little as 45° movement at the knees.
- Do not progress if you have knee pain in this exercise; limit deep knee bends.
- Inhalation on the downward phase helps to increase intra-abdominal pressure, keep the shoulders open, and prevent spinal flexion. Exhale on upward movement.

STARTING POSITION

- Take the bar off the squat rack safely and move back into a safe space for squatting.
- Press the bar directly overhead with elbows locked.
- Stand with your feet shoulder distance apart.
- Keep your posture aligned, with a neutral spine and knees soft.
- Hold bar wider than your shoulders, as is comfortable.
- Make sure your inner elbows are turned up toward the ceiling. Keep the shoulders back and down.

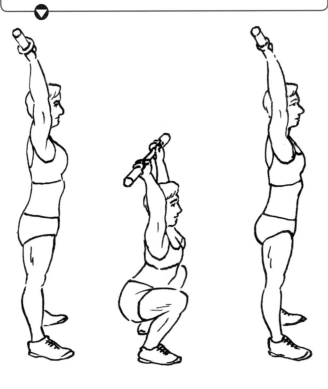

STABILIZING MUSCLES
• Abdominal group, Erector spinae, and Quadratus lumborum at the trunk
• Gluteus medius and minimus, Deep lateral rotators, and the Adductor group at the hips
• Ankle stabilizers and Gastrocnemius in the lower leg
• Rotator cuff muscles at the shoulder joint
• Serratus anterior, Rhomboids, and Lower trapezius at the shoulder blades
• Wrist flexors at the forearm

ANALYSIS OF MOVEMENT	JOINT 1	JOINT 2
Joints	Hip	Knee
Joint movement	Down – flexion Up – extension	Down – flexion Up – extension
Mobilizing muscles	Gluteus maximus Hamstring group	Quadricep group

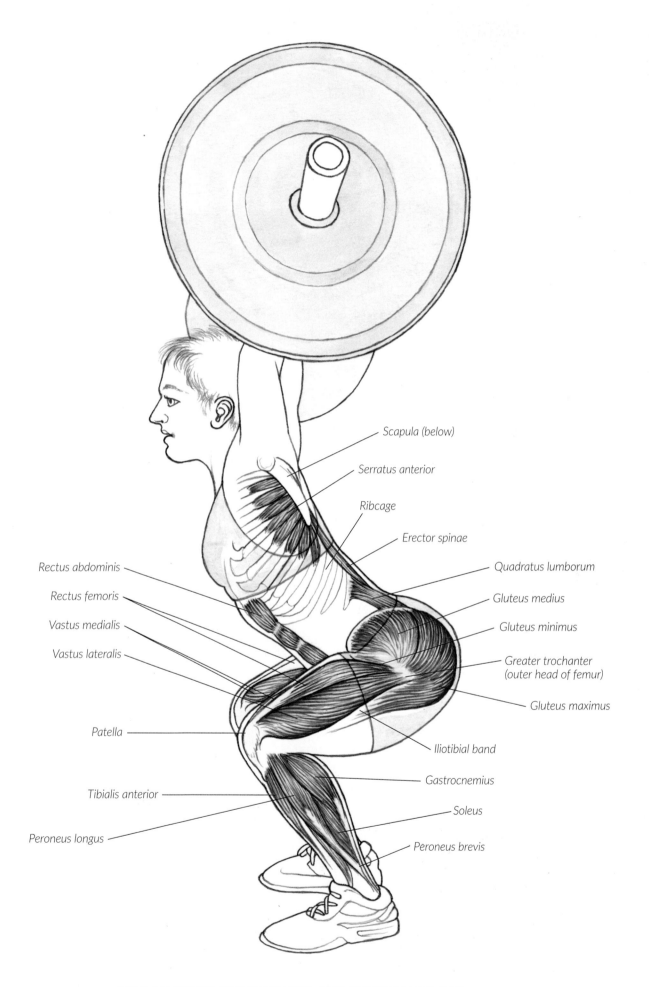

Scapula (below)

Serratus anterior

Ribcage

Erector spinae

Quadratus lumborum

Gluteus medius

Gluteus minimus

Greater trochanter
(outer head of femur)

Gluteus maximus

Iliotibial band

Gastrocnemius

Soleus

Peroneus brevis

Rectus abdominis

Rectus femoris

Vastus medialis

Vastus lateralis

Patella

Tibialis anterior

Peroneus longus

BARBELL STANDING SHOULDER PRESS

Core exercise• Compound/multi-joint • Push •
Close chain • Barbell • Intermediate to advanced

The barbell standing shoulder press is the functional foundation of all overhead lifts.

DESCRIPTION

Raise the barbell by extending the elbows. Lower to the upper chest. Repeat.

TRAINING TIPS

- Avoid momentum. Use a controlled, full range of movement.
- Once you achieve good form, you can increase to moderate velocity for more power emphasis.
- Avoid hunching or rounding the shoulders during the exercise. Keep the chest open and shoulder blades depressed.
- Brace and maintain the arch of the lumbar spine.
- Keep the heels down and drive through the heels and mid-foot.
- Core control and mindfulness are very important. Your core should be engaged to help with support and prevent injury.

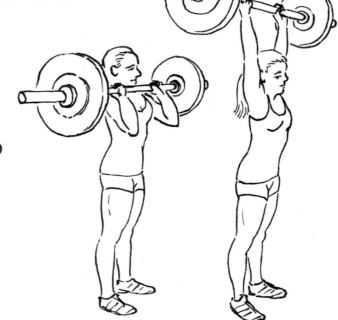

STARTING POSITION

- Stand with the feet shoulder-width apart.
- The barbell should be supported across the upper chest/shoulders.
- Place elbows below and in front of bar.
- Use an overhand grip, wider than shoulder-width.
- Keep the shoulders and chest open, elbows forward.
- Keep your posture aligned, with the spine neutral and stabilized.

ANALYSIS OF MOVEMENT	JOINT 1	JOINT 2	JOINT 3
Joints	Elbow	Shoulder	Scapulothoracic
Joint movement	Down – flexion Up – extension	Up – abduction, flexion Down – adduction, extension	Up – upward rotation Down – downward rotation
Mobilizing muscles	Triceps brachii Anconeus	Deltoid (emphasis on the anterior and mid fibers) Pectoralis major (clavicular aspect)	Serratus anterior Trapezius

STABILIZING MUSCLES

- All leg and hip muscles
- Abdominal group and Erector spinae at the trunk
- Rotator cuff muscles at the shoulder joint
- Serratus anterior, Rhomboids, and Lower trapezius at the shoulder blade
- Wrist flexors at the forearm

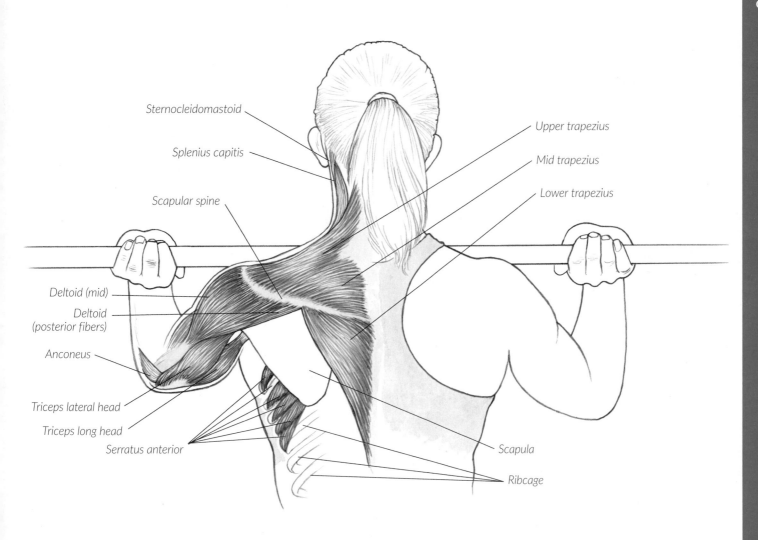

Sternocleidomastoid

Splenius capitis

Scapular spine

Deltoid (mid)

Deltoid
(posterior fibers)

Anconeus

Triceps lateral head

Triceps long head

Serratus anterior

Upper trapezius

Mid trapezius

Lower trapezius

Scapula

Ribcage

PUSH PRESS/PUSH JERK

Power exercises • Compound/multi-joint • Push
• Close chain • Barbell • Advanced

The push press and push jerk build on the shoulder press (see page 66). Though they have the same start and end positions and utilize the same muscles, the push jerk is not simply a press with extra help from the legs.

DESCRIPTION

The start position for the push press and push jerk are the same. So, too, are the end position, path of the bar, and the initial dip and drive of the legs. The essential difference is that in the push press, the dip, drive, and press follow one synchronized motion, with the press being a continuous part of the lift. In a push press, your arms press the weight overhead. In the push jerk, on the other hand, with the initial dip and drive, as your arms press upward against the bar, it pushes the hips and knees back into a second dip. From there, the knees and hip extensors then drive the bar upwards to its end position.

STARTING POSITION

- Stand with your feet shoulder-width apart.
- Support the barbell across the upper chest with a shoulder-width overhand grip.
- Keep your shoulders and chest open, with elbows forward.
- Keep your posture aligned and stabilized.
- Note: The starting position is the same as the end position for the power clean (see page 76).

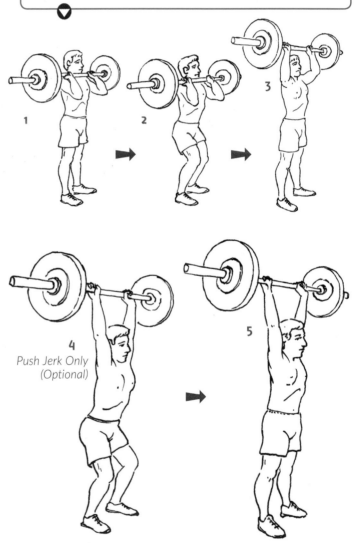

PUSH PRESS
From the start position, lower your body into a quarter squat
With rebound momentum, explosively drive the bar upward, with the legs extending at the knee and hip.
Continue the momentum through the arms and shoulders to press the bar upward into its overhead position, fully extending the elbows.
Keep your heels down as the legs extend.
Complete the full hip, knee, and elbow extension.
Return the bar to your shoulders and repeat.
Throughout the movement, maintain the bar balanced over the mid-foot.
Short cues are dip, drive, press.
Emphasis is on arm and shoulder power development.

PUSH JERK
From the start position, lower your body into a quarter squat
With rebound momentum, drive upward from the hip and knee while the arms press up against the bar.
This initiates a second dip in the hip and knees so that the bar is received in a partial squat position. Drive the bar upward again, by extending your knees and hips.
Keep your heels down as the legs extend.
Complete the full hip, knee, and elbow extension.
Return the bar to your shoulders and repeat.
Throughout the movement, maintain the bar balanced over the mid-foot.
Short cues are dip, drive, press and dip, drive.
Emphasis is on leg and hip power development.

Push Jerk Only (Optional)

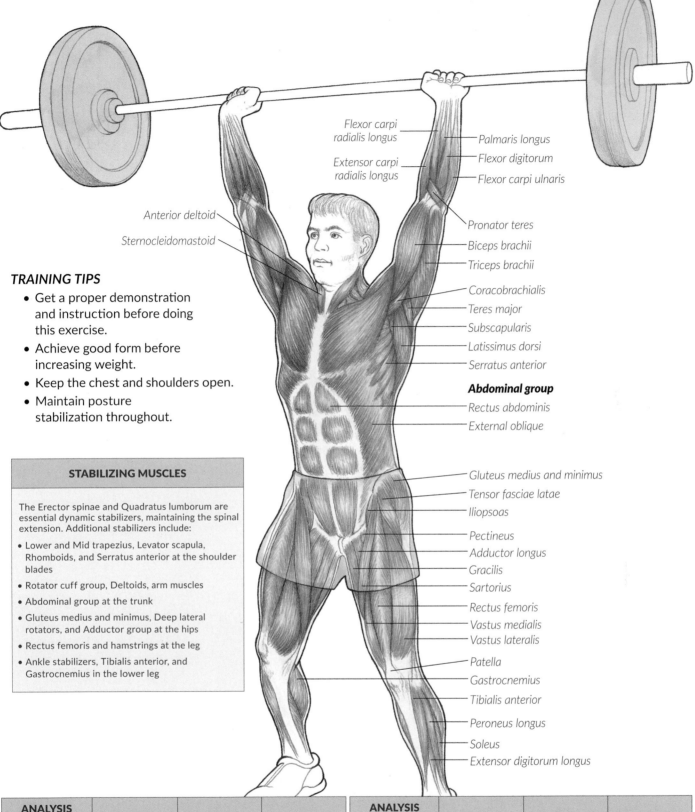

Flexor carpi radialis longus
Extensor carpi radialis longus
Palmaris longus
Flexor digitorum
Flexor carpi ulnaris
Anterior deltoid
Sternocleidomastoid
Pronator teres
Biceps brachii
Triceps brachii
Coracobrachialis
Teres major
Subscapularis
Latissimus dorsi
Serratus anterior
Abdominal group
Rectus abdominis
External oblique
Gluteus medius and minimus
Tensor fasciae latae
Iliopsoas
Pectineus
Adductor longus
Gracilis
Sartorius
Rectus femoris
Vastus medialis
Vastus lateralis
Patella
Gastrocnemius
Tibialis anterior
Peroneus longus
Soleus
Extensor digitorum longus

TRAINING TIPS

- Get a proper demonstration and instruction before doing this exercise.
- Achieve good form before increasing weight.
- Keep the chest and shoulders open.
- Maintain posture stabilization throughout.

STABILIZING MUSCLES

The Erector spinae and Quadratus lumborum are essential dynamic stabilizers, maintaining the spinal extension. Additional stabilizers include:

- Lower and Mid trapezius, Levator scapula, Rhomboids, and Serratus anterior at the shoulder blades
- Rotator cuff group, Deltoids, arm muscles
- Abdominal group at the trunk
- Gluteus medius and minimus, Deep lateral rotators, and Adductor group at the hips
- Rectus femoris and hamstrings at the leg
- Ankle stabilizers, Tibialis anterior, and Gastrocnemius in the lower leg

ANALYSIS OF MOVEMENT LOWER BODY	JOINT 1	JOINT 2	JOINT 3
Joints	Ankle	Knee	Hip
Joint movement	Up – plantarflexion	Up – extension	Up – extension
Mobilizing muscles	Gastrocnemius Soleus	Quadricep group	Gluteus maximus Hamstring group

ANALYSIS OF MOVEMENT UPPER BODY	JOINT 4	JOINT 5	JOINT 6
Joints	Elbow	Shoulder	Scapulothoracic
Joint movement	Up – extension	Up – flexion, abduction	Up – upward rotation
Mobilizing muscles	Triceps brachii Anconeus	Anterior and Mid deltoid Pectoralis major (clavicular aspect)	Serratus anterior

Note: For the purpose of simplicity, we have only detailed the active phase (i.e., the up phase) of the exercise.

NEW ANATOMY FOR STRENGTH AND FITNESS TRAINING

BARBELL BENT LEG DEAD LIFT

Core exercise • Compound/multi-joint
• Pull • Close chain • Barbell
• Intermediate to advanced

The dead lift, one of the most complete exercises, is one of three events in competitive powerlifting (alongside the bench press and squat). The aim is to lift the heaviest weight possible. The dead lift has a place in functional training and back rehabilitation regimes, and is an ideal preparation for the power clean and jerk.

DESCRIPTION

Lift the bar by extending the knees and hips, using the combined strength of the back, hips, and thighs. Return and repeat.

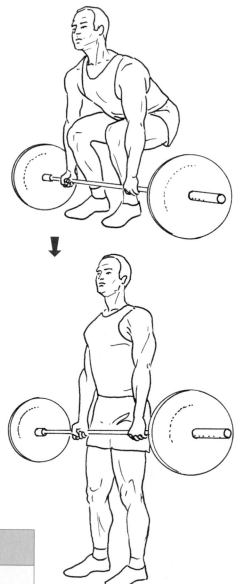

STARTING POSITION

- Stand with feet shoulder-width apart and underneath the barbell.
- Squat down and grasp the bar with an alternate over-grip (one hand over, one hand under).
- Grip width is shoulder-width or slightly wider.
- Keep posture aligned.

TRAINING TIPS

- Get a proper demonstration and instruction before doing this exercise.
- Establish good form before increasing weight.
- In the lift, lead with the head and shoulders; keep the hips low.
- Once the bar passes the knee, push the hips forward.
- Throughout the exercise, keep the bar close to the body.
- Try to keep the chest and shoulders open.
- Maintain posture stabilization throughout.
- Inhaling on the upward phase helps to increase intra-abdominal pressure, keep the shoulders open, and prevent spinal flexion. Exhale on the downward movement.

ANALYSIS OF MOVEMENT	JOINT 1	JOINT 2	JOINT 3
Joints	Knee	Hip	Spine
Joint movement	Up – extension Down – flexion	Up – extension Down – flexion	Up – extension Down – flexion to neutral
Mobilizing muscles	Quadricep group	Gluteus maximus Hamstring group	Erector spinae

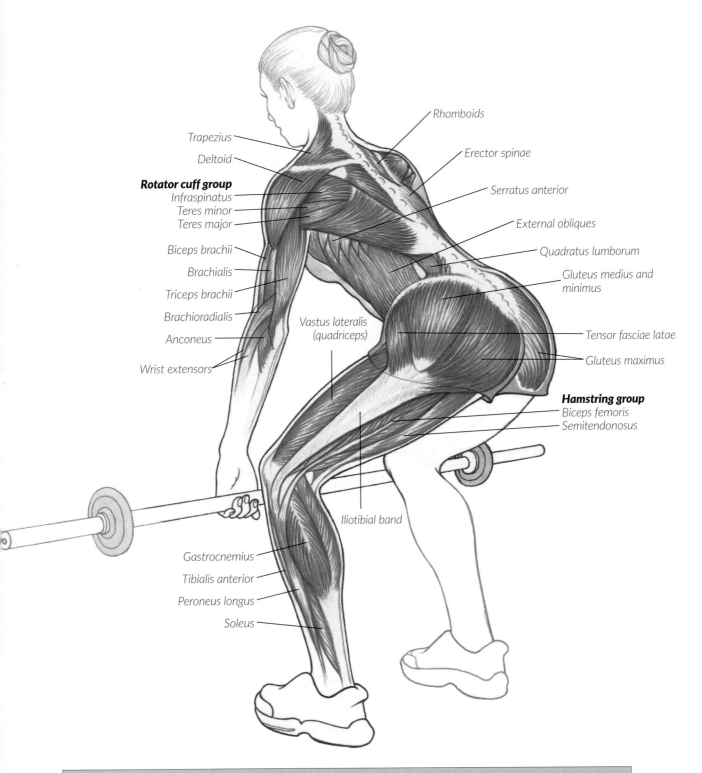

Rhomboids

Trapezius

Deltoid

Erector spinae

Rotator cuff group
Infraspinatus
Teres minor
Teres major

Serratus anterior

External obliques

Quadratus lumborum

Biceps brachii

Brachialis

Triceps brachii

Gluteus medius and minimus

Brachioradialis

Vastus lateralis
(quadriceps)

Anconeus

Tensor fasciae latae

Wrist extensors

Gluteus maximus

Hamstring group
Biceps femoris
Semitendonosus

Iliotibial band

Gastrocnemius

Tibialis anterior

Peroneus longus

Soleus

STABILIZING MUSCLES

The Erector spinae and Quadratus lumborum are essential dynamic stabilizers, maintaining the spinal extension. Additional stabilizers include:

- Shoulder blades: Lower and Mid trapezius, Levator scapula, Rhomboids, Serratus anterior
- Arm muscles: Rotator cuff group, Deltoids, Biceps, Triceps, forearm muscles
- Trunk: Abdominal group
- Hips: Gluteus medius and minimus, Deep external hip rotators, Adductor group
- Lower leg: Ankle stabilizers, Tibialis anterior, Gastrocnemius

MEDICINE BALL CLEAN

Core exercise • Compound/multi-joint • Push • Close chain • Medicine ball • Intermediate to advanced

Regarded as one of the most complex of the 9 basic movements of CrossFit, the medicine ball clean builds on the foundations of the dead lift and the sumo high pull. In itself, it is a great foundational exercise and can help develop form for the dead lift, clean, and snatch lifts.

DESCRIPTION

From the squat position, accelerate upward, extending at the hips and knees, pulling the ball upward. The momentum carries into a shoulder shrug. At the top end of the shrug, the trunks dips down into a deep squat, as the arms pull under the ball, "catching" it in front of the face/upper chest. Accelerate upward, extending the hips and knees fully. Return and repeat.

STARTING POSITION

- Get into squat position.
- With your heels flat, keep your knees vertically in line with the toes, and the feet shoulder distance apart.
- Keep your posture aligned with a neutral spine, eyes looking slightly above horizon.
- Hold the ball between your feet.

TRAINING TIPS

- Achieve good form before increasing ball weight.
- Use controlled momentum.
- When lifting, keep the ball close to the body; the ball keeps the arms locked.
- Keep the elbows high when "catching" the ball.
- Brace and maintain the arch of the lumbar spine.
- Don't drop the head; maintain eye level just above horizontal with neutral cervical spine.
- Keep your chest open, avoiding rounding the shoulders.
- Keep the knees from passing over the vertical line of the toes.
- Keep your weight directly over the heel to mid-foot. Avoid lifting the heels.
- If there are joint or injury limitations at knee, only go down to 90° (keep hips above knees in the squat).

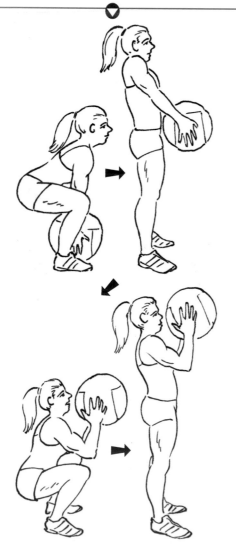

ANALYSIS OF MOVEMENT	JOINT 1	JOINT 2	JOINT 3
PHASE 1: Squat Position, up to Shrug (Concentric Phase)			
Joints	Hip	Knee	Spine
Joint movement	Up – extension	Up – extension	Up – extension
Mobilizing muscles	Gluteus maximus Hamstring group	Quadricep group	Erector spinae
Joints	Shoulders	Scapula	
Joint movement	Up – flexion, abduction, lateral rotation	Up – elevation, upward rotation	
Mobilizing muscles	Deltoid Supraspinatus Infraspinatus Teres minor Pectoralis major (clavicular aspect)	Upper trapezius Levator scapula Serratus anterior	
PHASE 2: Shrug, down to Deep Squat (Eccentric Phase)			
Joints	Hip	Knee	Elbow
Joint movement	Down – flexion	Down – flexion	Down – flexion
Mobilizing muscles	Gluteus maximus Hamstring group	Quadricep group	Biceps brachii Brachialis Brachoradialis
PHASE 3: Deep Squat, up to Standing Position (Concentric Phase)			
Joints	Hip	Knee	
Joint movement	Up – extension	Up – extension	
Mobilizing muscles	Gluteus maximus Hamstring group	Quadricep group	

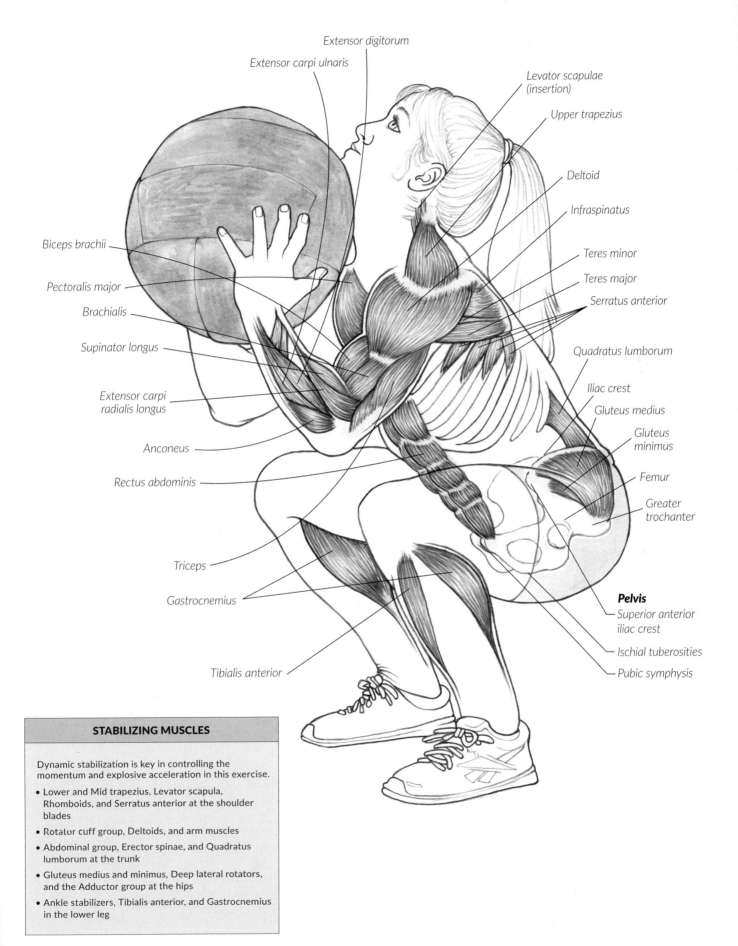

Extensor digitorum

Extensor carpi ulnaris

Levator scapulae (insertion)

Upper trapezius

Deltoid

Infraspinatus

Biceps brachii

Teres minor

Teres major

Serratus anterior

Pectoralis major

Brachialis

Quadratus lumborum

Supinator longus

Iliac crest

Gluteus medius

Extensor carpi radialis longus

Gluteus minimus

Femur

Anconeus

Greater trochanter

Rectus abdominis

Pelvis
Superior anterior iliac crest

Triceps

Ischial tuberosities

Gastrocnemius

Pubic symphysis

Tibialis anterior

STABILIZING MUSCLES

Dynamic stabilization is key in controlling the momentum and explosive acceleration in this exercise.

- Lower and Mid trapezius, Levator scapula, Rhomboids, and Serratus anterior at the shoulder blades
- Rotator cuff group, Deltoids, and arm muscles
- Abdominal group, Erector spinae, and Quadratus lumborum at the trunk
- Gluteus medius and minimus, Deep lateral rotators, and the Adductor group at the hips
- Ankle stabilizers, Tibialis anterior, and Gastrocnemius in the lower leg

SUMO DEAD LIFT HIGH PULL

Core exercise • Compound/multi-joint • Pull •
Close chain • Barbell • Advanced

This explosive exercise builds on the dead lift, adding velocity with a wider stance for stability.

DESCRIPTION

Lift the bar by extending the knees and hips, using the strength of the back, hips, and thighs. Let the hips extend fully, transferring momentum into the arms and shoulders, into a shrug. Keeping elbows above the hands, pull the bar right up under the chin. Return and repeat.

TRAINING TIPS

- Get a proper demonstration and instruction before doing this exercise.
- Achieve good form before increasing weight.
- In the lift, lead with the head, keeping eyes forward.
- Once the bar passes the knee, continue to extend the hips forward.
- Keep the heels down.
- Throughout the exercise, keep the bar close to the body, elbows always higher than hands.
- Brace and maintain the arch of the lumbar spine.
- Avoid hunching or rounding the shoulders. Keep the chest open and shoulder blades depressed and retracted.
- Maintain posture stabilization and lumbar brace throughout.

STARTING POSITION

- Place feet wider than shoulder-width, feet 45° outwardly rotated.
- With heels flat, keep the knees vertically in line with the toes.
- Squat down and grasp the bar with an over-grip.
- Keep a close grip on the bar, with shoulders slightly forward of the bar and posture aligned.

STABILIZING MUSCLES

The Erector spinae and Quadratus lumborum are essential dynamic stabilizers, maintaining the spinal extension. Additional stabilizers involved include:

- Lower and Mid trapezius, Levator scapula, Rhomboids, and Serratus anterior at the shoulder blades
- Rotator cuff group, Posterior deltoids
- Abdominal group at the trunk
- Gluteus medius and minimus, Deep lateral rotators, and Adductor group at the hips
- Ankle stabilizers, Tibialis anterior, and Gastrocnemius in the lower leg

ANALYSIS OF MOVEMENT	JOINT 1	JOINT 2	JOINT 3
Joints	Knee	Hip	Spine
Joint movement	Up – extension, some adduction Down – flexion, some abduction	Up – extension Down – flexion	Up – extension Down – flexion, back to neutral
Mobilizing muscles	Quadricep group Adductor group	Gluteus maximus Hamstring group	Erector spinae

	JOINT 4	JOINT 5	JOINT 6
Joints	Elbow	Shoulder	Scapulothoracic
Joint movement	Up – flexion Down – extension	Up – abduction, medial rotation Down – adduction, lateral rotation	Up – upward rotation Down – downward rotation
Mobilizing muscles	Bicep brachii Brachialis Brachoradialis	Deltoid (emphasis on anterior and lateral aspect)	Trapezius Rhomboids Serratus anterior

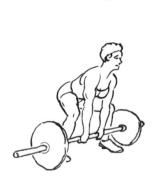
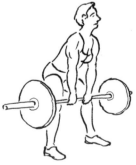
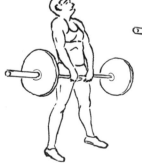
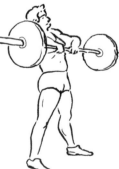
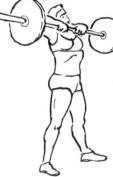

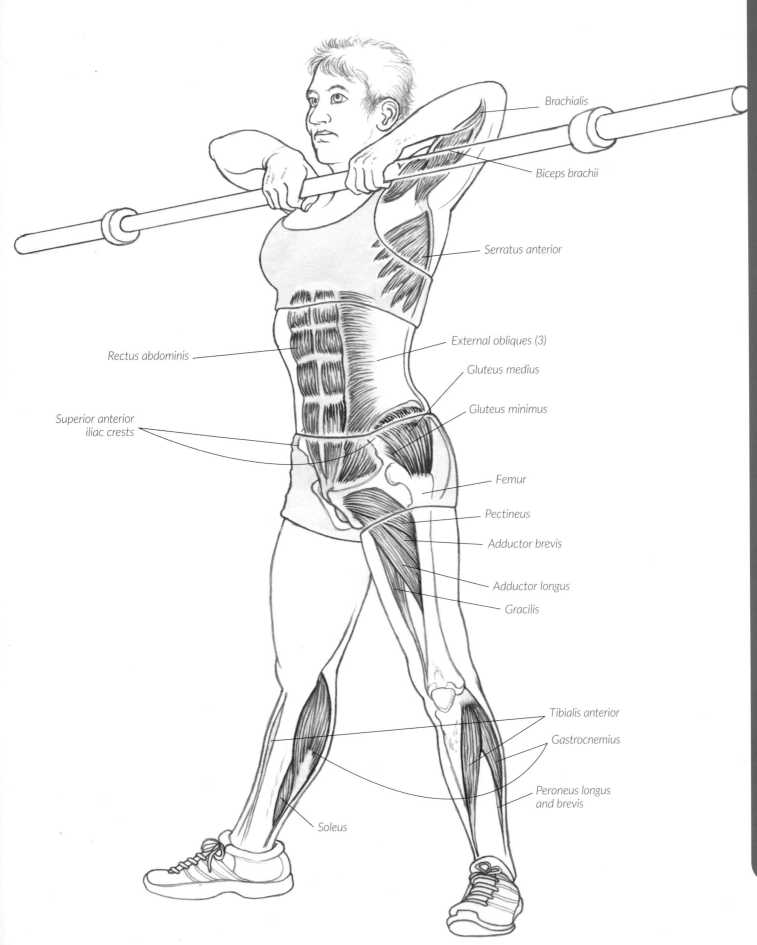

Brachialis

Biceps brachii

Serratus anterior

Rectus abdominis

External obliques (3)

Gluteus medius

Gluteus minimus

Superior anterior
iliac crests

Femur

Pectineus

Adductor brevis

Adductor longus

Gracilis

Tibialis anterior

Gastrocnemius

Peroneus longus
and brevis

Soleus

NEW ANATOMY FOR STRENGTH AND FITNESS TRAINING

POWER CLEAN

Power exercise • Compound/multi-joint •
Pull • Close chain • Barbell • Advanced

The power clean forms the first phase of the clean and jerk. You should master the individual phases before combining them into one exercise.

DESCRIPTION

Pull the bar up off the floor by extending the hips and knees. Using the upward momentum, as the bar reaches the knees, explosively raise the shoulders, keeping the barbell close to the thighs.

When the barbell reaches mid-thigh, jump upward and thrust the hips forward, extending the body. This will accelerate the upward momentum of the bar. At this point, most of the work shifts from the legs and lower back to the upper back, shoulders, and arms.

As the bar moves past waist height, pull the body underneath the bar, bending the elbows, and drop down onto a flat foot, so that you end in a half squat, with the barbell supported on the upper chest and the elbows pointing forward. Stand up and stabilize.

Return by dropping the elbows and controlling the bar down to mid-thigh. From there, squat down to the starting position.

TRAINING TIPS

- Get a proper demonstration and qualified instruction.
- Establish good form before increasing weight.
- In the lift, lead with the head and shoulders.
- Do not jerk the weight: rise steadily, then accelerate. Generate the power into the legs and back, and then shift it fluidly to the upper back, shoulders, and arms.
- Throughout the exercise, keep the bar close to the body.
- Maintain posture stabilization throughout.
- Inhaling on the upward phase helps to increase intra-abdominal pressure, keep the shoulders open, and prevent spinal flexion.

STARTING POSITION

- Stand with your feet shoulder-width apart beneath the barbell.
- Squat down and grasp the bar with an overhand grip, slightly wider than shoulder-width.
- Pull the shoulders back so they are positioned over the bar.
- Arch your back slightly, pushing the buttocks back.
- Extend the arms.
- Keep your posture aligned and stabilized.

ANALYSIS OF MOVEMENT	JOINT 1	JOINT 2	JOINT 3	JOINT 4
Joints	Ankle	Knee	Hip	Spine
Joint movement	Up – plantarflexion	Up – extension	Up – extension	Up – extension
Mobilizing muscles	Gastrocnemius Soleus	Quadricep group	Gluteus maximus Hamstring group	Erector spinae

	JOINT 5	JOINT 6	JOINT 7	JOINT 8
Joints	Shoulders	Scapula	Elbow	Wrist
Joint movement	Up – flexion, abduction, external rotation	Up – elevation, Upward rotation	Up – flexion	Up – extension
Mobilizing muscles	Deltoid, Supraspinatus, Infraspinatus, Teres minor Pectoralis major (clavicular aspect)	Upper trapezius Levator scapula Serratus anterior	Bicep group	Extensor carpi radialis longus Extensor carpi radialis brevis Extensor carpi ulnaris

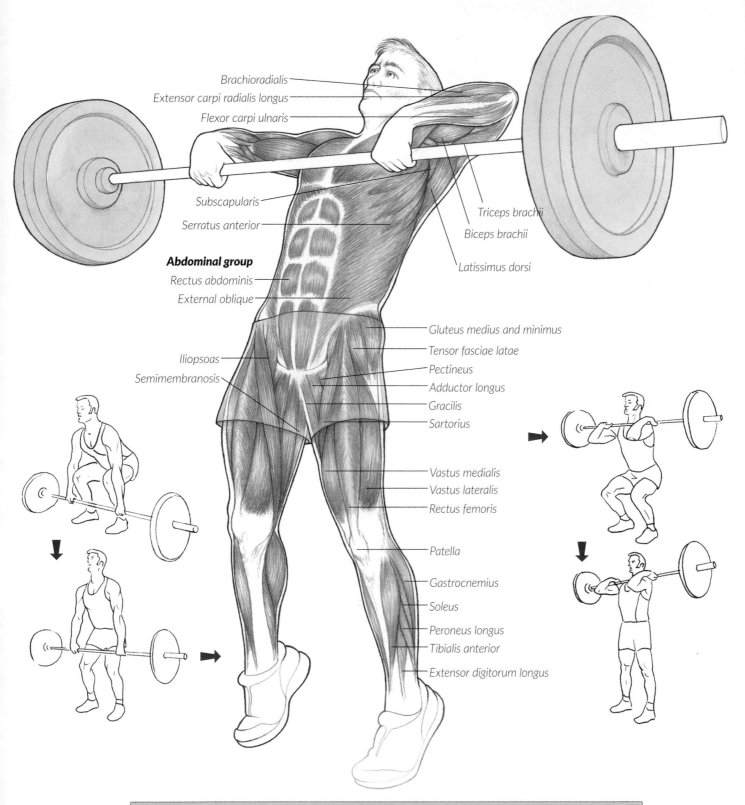

Brachioradialis
Extensor carpi radialis longus
Flexor carpi ulnaris
Subscapularis
Serratus anterior
Abdominal group
Rectus abdominis
External oblique
Iliopsoas
Semimembranosis
Triceps brachii
Biceps brachii
Latissimus dorsi
Gluteus medius and minimus
Tensor fasciae latae
Pectineus
Adductor longus
Gracilis
Sartorius
Vastus medialis
Vastus lateralis
Rectus femoris
Patella
Gastrocnemius
Soleus
Peroneus longus
Tibialis anterior
Extensor digitorum longus

STABILIZING MUSCLES

The Erector spinae and Quadratus lumborum are essential dynamic stabilizers, maintaining the spinal extension. Additional stabilizers include:

- Shoulder blades: Lower and Mid trapezius, Levator scapula, Rhomboids, Serratus anterior
- Arms: Rotator cuff group, Deltoids, arm muscles
- Trunk: Abdominal group
- Hips: Gluteus group, deep external hip rotators, Adductor group
- Legs: Rectus femoris, Hamstrings
- Lower legs: Ankle stabilizers, Tibialis anterior, Gastrocnemius

POWER SNATCH

*Power exercise • Compound/multi-joint • Pull •
Close chain • Barbell • Advanced*

The appropriately named snatch is a fast, synchronized lift that requires timing, muscle coordination, good conditioning, and excellent stability. It is a high-risk exercise, not to be practiced without proper instruction and supervision.

DESCRIPTION

Stand with your feet shoulder-width apart, underneath the barbell. Squat down and grasp the bar with an overhand grip, roughly double your shoulder-width. Pull the shoulders back until they are positioned over the bar. Arch the back slightly, pushing the buttocks back, and keep the arms extended.

TRAINING TIPS

- Achieve good form before increasing weight.
- In the lift, lead with the head and shoulders.
- The snatch needs to be one coordinated, continuous movement executed with speed. Do not jerk the weight from the floor. Rise steadily, then accelerate. Generate power into the legs and back, and shift it fluidly to the upper back, shoulders, and arms.
- Maintain posture stabilization throughout.
- Inhale on the upward phase to help increase intra-abdominal pressure, keep the shoulders open, and prevent spinal flexion.

ANALYSIS OF MOVEMENT	JOINT 1	JOINT 2	JOINT 3	JOINT 4
Joints	Ankle	Knee	Hip	Spine
Joint movement	Up – plantarflexion	Up – extension	Up – extension	Up – extension
Mobilizing muscles	Gastrocnemius Soleus	Quadricep group	Gluteus maximus Hamstring group	Erector spinae

	JOINT 5	JOINT 6	JOINT 7	JOINT 8
Joints	Shoulders	Scapula	Elbow	Wrist
Joint movement	Up – flexion, abduction, external rotation	Up – elevation Upward rotation	Up – extension	Up – extension
Mobilizing muscles	Deltoid Supraspinatus Infraspinatus Teres minor Pectoralis major (clavicular aspect)	Upper trapezius Levator scapula Serratus anterior	Tricep brachii Anconeus	Extensor carpi radialis longus Extensor carpi radialis brevis Extensor carpi ulnaris

STABILIZING MUSCLES	The Erector spinae and Quadratus lumborum maintain spinal extension. • Shoulder blades: Lower and mid-Trapezius, Levator scapula, Rhomboids, Serratus anterior • Arms: Rotator cuff group (very important), Deltoids, arm muscles • Trunk: Abdominal group • Hips: Gluteus medius and minimus, deep external hip rotators, Adductor group • Legs: Rectus femoris, Hamstring group • Lower leg: Ankle stabilizers, Tibialis anterior, Gastrocnemius

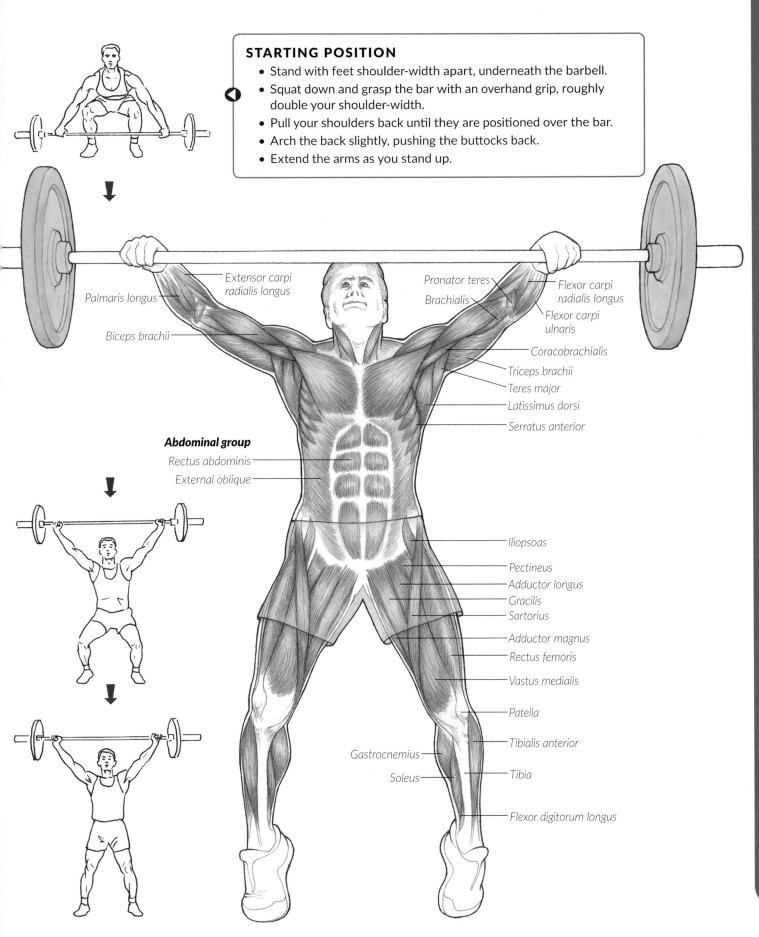

STARTING POSITION
- Stand with feet shoulder-width apart, underneath the barbell.
- Squat down and grasp the bar with an overhand grip, roughly double your shoulder-width.
- Pull your shoulders back until they are positioned over the bar.
- Arch the back slightly, pushing the buttocks back.
- Extend the arms as you stand up.

Palmaris longus

Extensor carpi radialis longus

Biceps brachii

Pronator teres

Brachialis

Flexor carpi radialis longus

Flexor carpi ulnaris

Coracobrachialis

Triceps brachii

Teres major

Latissimus dorsi

Serratus anterior

Abdominal group

Rectus abdominis

External oblique

Iliopsoas

Pectineus

Adductor longus

Gracilis

Sartorius

Adductor magnus

Rectus femoris

Vastus medialis

Patella

Tibialis anterior

Gastrocnemius

Tibia

Soleus

Flexor digitorum longus

NEW ANATOMY FOR STRENGTH AND FITNESS TRAINING

LOW ALTERNATING WAVE WITH BATTLE ROPES

Compound • Close chain • Battle ropes •
Intermediate to advanced

The low alternating wave is an entry-level battle rope exercise that can help establish the speed, stabilization, and control required when working with battle ropes.

BATTLE ROPE ESSENTIALS

American John Brookfield holds multiple impressive world records in a range of strength feats. In the early 2000s, as part of his training, he began experimenting in his backyard with heavy ropes as a training tool for increased power endurance. He later formalized this into a training system, Battling Ropes®, which became popular with performance athletes. The use of ropes has since spread as a training tool into CrossFit and functional gyms alike.

Battle ropes come in a variety of types, thicknesses, and lengths, with the 50-foot-long, 1-inch-wide (15m-long, 2.5cm-wide) rope being the most common. Weight and difficulty increase with increasing thickness and length. Ropes are made from nylon or polyester/polypropylene as well as the original manila material, which tends to fray more than its synthetic counterparts.

When training, the rope is wrapped around an anchor point, and you hold it at the very end of the rope's length. You can do partner workouts with either person holding one end of the rope. By holding the rope with an overhand grip or an underhand grip, you initiate and maintain a whipping or circular motion with your arms, creating a wave motion in the rope that requires a constant metabolic work to maintain.

Battle rope workouts have some unique features.

First, with battle ropes, you cannot leverage momentum and gravity to aid movement, like you can with dumbbells, barbells, and kettlebells. Instead, you must constantly generate and maintain velocity to complete the exercise. Stabilization also has to be constant. This increases the work rate and total overload of the exercise. As a result, battle ropes are one of the more effective forms of power endurance training. This places intense, short-term demand on the energy systems of the body.

Second, in most barbell, dumbbell, and kettlebell exercises, you have a concentric and eccentric phase for the main muscles working (which we call the agonists). In the concentric phase, the muscle shortens under load, and in the eccentric phase, it lengthens under load. However, with battle ropes, both the agonist and antagonist (i.e., opposing

STARTING POSITION

- Stand facing the anchor point of the battle rope.
- Grab one end of the rope in each hand so that your palms face in.
- Stand with feet shoulder distance apart, and lower into the squat position.
- Keep posture aligned and stabilized.
- Activate your stabilizing muscles to maintain stable posture and lumbar curve.

Sternocleidomastoid
Upper trapezius
Deltoid
Teres major
Teres minor
Triceps
Latissimus dorsi
Serratus anterior
Gluteus medius
Gluteus maximus
External obliques
Vastus lateralis
Tibialis anterior

Pectoralis major
Deltoid
Biceps
Rectus abdominis
Rectus femoris
Vastus medialis
Gastrocnemius
Soleus

Battle Rope Essentials (continued)

muscles) go through concentric phases, having to actively contract to move the ropes in both directions.

Third, the slack you allow in the rope will determine intensity. The closer you move to the anchor point, the more resistance you'll be creating as you are forced to generate more power to make the waves reach the anchor point, thus also increasing overload. Moving away from the anchor point decreases exercise intensity.

Most basic battle rope movements incorporate wave, slam, and whipping motions, and can incorporate compound movements like squats, lunges, and jumps. While they train mostly upper body power and mobilization, battle ropes tax the full range of core and joint stabilizers and have a training effect on aerobic endurance.

As a typical rule, changing the variables of training and rest changes the training effect and outcome. Here are some examples. For peak strength, use 10–20 seconds of movement with 20–60 seconds of rest. For muscle growth, use 20–60 seconds of movement with 40–120 seconds of rest. For strength endurance, use 60–120 seconds of movement with 60–20 seconds of rest.

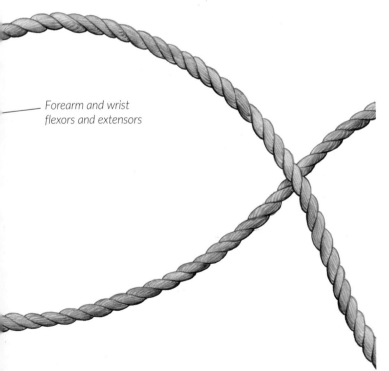

Forearm and wrist flexors and extensors

DESCRIPTION

Using rapid, controlled movement, raise and lower your arms in an alternating pattern to cause an undulating wave in the rope.

STABILIZING MUSCLES
The Erector spinae and Quadratus lumborum are essential dynamic stabilizers, maintaining the spinal extension. Additional stabilizers involved include:
• Lower and Mid trapezius, Levator scapula, Rhomboids, and Serratus anterior at the shoulder blades
• Rotator cuff group, Posterior deltoids
• Abdominal group at the trunk
• Gluteus medius and minimus, Deep lateral rotators, and Adductor group at the hips
• Ankle stabilizers, Tibialis anterior, and Gastrocnemius in the lower leg
• Wrist extensors at the forearm

ANALYSIS OF MOVEMENT	JOINT 1
Joints	Shoulder
Joint movement	Up – flexion Down – extension
Mobilizing muscles	Deltoid (emphasis on the anterior aspect on the way up, posterior aspect on the way down) Latissimus dorsi Pectoralis major (emphasis on the clavicular aspect on the way up, pectoral aspect on the way down)

Technical point: *On the upward movement, the shoulder flexors are working concentrically; on the downward movement, the shoulders extensors are working concentrically.*

TRAINING TIPS

- It is key to maintain stabilization for the duration of the exercise in order to generate maximum power output.
- Let the shoulders generate movements; the trunk and legs muscles anchor your body.
- Avoid rounding the chest and hunching the shoulders. Keep them open. Aim to depress and widen the shoulder blades against the back, activating the Serratus anterior.
- For beginners, scale back the exercise by reducing the squat, standing with soft knees, while still maintaining postural stabilization. Beginners can also stand further away from the anchor point.

KETTLEBELL SWING

Compound • Close chain • Kettlebell • Beginner to advanced

The kettlebell swing is shown here in its original Russian version and its adapted American counterpart. The exercise has applications to warm-up, speed/power, strength, posture, and HIIT training.

KETTLEBELL ESSENTIALS

The kettlebell, originally called a girya, first began to appear in Russia in the 18th century, where farmers used it to weigh grains. Soon the farmers began challenging each other to feats of strength using the girya. By 1885, this had developed into a sport called girevoy, which became a formalized sport in 1970. The kettlebell also made its way into the circus strongman culture popular in the late 19th century, and by the 1940s had made its way to the United States, where it became known as a kettlebell.

Russian kettlebells were traditionally measured in the standards of the Russian imperial weight system. In that now-obsolete system, a pood, equivalent to 36.1 lbs (16.38kg), was the standard weight unit for girya. In current kettlebell exercise, men usually start training with a kettlebell of 15–25 lbs (7–11kg), whereas women usually start with a kettlebell of 8–15 lbs (3–7kg).

The kettlebell design is unique. It comprises a bell, handle, and horns; the bell is the round weight, and the handle connects to the bell by the sloping downward horns on each side. Unlike a dumbbell, a kettlebell's center of gravity is offset from its handle. This means that the load of the kettlebell lies 6–8 in (15–20cm) away from your grip on the handle, making it harder to control than a dumbbell. This increases the stabilization requirement of the muscles in a given exercise. The kettlebell is also less forgiving if your form and core stability are off, as its center of gravity will pull you in the direction of your imbalance and poor form.

(continued on facing page)

DESCRIPTION

RUSSIAN:
The kettlebell is swung up to chest level, using an efficient rhythm generated from hip joint movement.

AMERICAN:
The kettlebell is swung to directly overhead, using an efficient rhythm generated from hip joint movement.

TRAINING TIPS

- The American kettlebell swing only differs from the traditional Russian swing in the top position. The start position and movement pattern of the swing itself are identical.
- The power of the swing is generated from the hip extensors, while the spine is held perfectly stable and neutral.
- The key to a good kettlebell swing is effectively generating the controlled momentum at the hips and sending the weight forwards, as opposed to squatting the weight up or lifting up with the arms. This requires an intense stabilization while generating power primarily from the Glutes and secondarily from the shoulder muscles.
- In the American swing, do not elevate the shoulders to raise the kettlebell into the top position.
- Avoid rounding the chest and hunching the shoulders. Keep them open. Aim to depress and widen the shoulder blades against the back, activating the Serratus anterior.
- While the American version of the swing moves the kettlebell through a greater range of motion, it places mores stress on the relatively unstable shoulder joint at the top portion of the swing. Therefore, in the American swing, use a relatively lower weight compared to the Russian swing.
- Choose a weight that allows proper form and the strength or speed/power outcome desired (i.e., heavier weights for strength, moderately lighter for speed and power).
- Inhale on the downward swing motion, exhale at the top of the swing.

STARTING POSITION ▶

- Stand with your feet shoulder distance apart.
- Keep your posture aligned and your spine neutral.
- Knees should be at approximately 30° flexion.
- Keep elbows extended with a firm grip on the kettlebell, held just in front of the body.
- Note: Both the Russian and American swing have the same starting position.

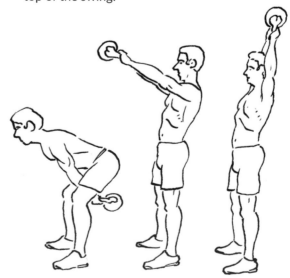

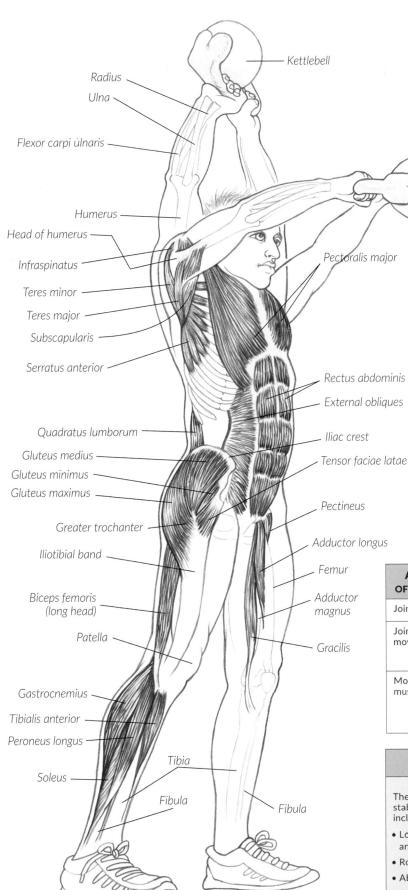

Radius
Ulna
Flexor carpi ülnaris
Humerus
Head of humerus
Infraspinatus
Teres minor
Teres major
Subscapularis
Serratus anterior
Quadratus lumborum
Gluteus medius
Gluteus minimus
Gluteus maximus
Greater trochanter
Iliotibial band
Biceps femoris (long head)
Patella
Gastrocnemius
Tibialis anterior
Peroneus longus
Soleus
Tibia
Fibula

Kettlebell
Pectoralis major
Rectus abdominis
External obliques
Iliac crest
Tensor faciae latae
Pectineus
Adductor longus
Femur
Adductor magnus
Gracilis
Fibula

The kettlebell can be a standalone exercise training option and is ideal for home training. It's also widely used as part of CrossFit, HIIT, functional, and martial arts training programs. The offset center of gravity in a kettlebell facilitates ballistic and swinging movements. This, in turn, lends kettlebells to compound training, working multiple muscle groups simultaneously, with higher repetition and endurance components and higher demand on stabilization muscle work. Many of the typical compound exercises found in this book have a kettlebell version counterpart. Exercises such as the swing, snatch, clean and jerk, push press, overhead squat, dead lift, lunge, and row are standard in kettlebell programs.

As always, good form should be trained and maintained to ensure safe and effective overload. When executed properly, kettlebell work offers improved posture, greater range of motion, and increased strength. As a general rule, higher weights and lower repetitions offer more of a strength stimulus, while relatively lower weights and higher speeds offer more speed stimulus. Increased repetitions offer more aerobic conditioning.

ANALYSIS OF MOVEMENT	JOINT 1	JOINT 2
Joints	Shoulder	Hip
Joint movement	Up – flexion Down – extension	Up – extension Down – flexion
Mobilizing muscles	Deltoid (emphasis on the anterior aspect) Pectoralis major (emphasis on clavicular aspect)	Gluteus maximus Hamstring group

STABILIZING MUSCLES

The Erector spinae and Quadratus lumborum are essential dynamic stabilizers, maintaining the spinal extension. Additional stabilizers involved include:

• Lower and Mid trapezius, Levator scapula, Rhomboids, and Serratus anterior at the shoulder blades
• Rotator cuff group, Posterior deltoids
• Abdominal group at the trunk
• Gluteus medius and minimus, Deep lateral rotators, and Adductor group at the hips
• Ankle stabilizers, Tibialis anterior, and Gastrocnemius in the lower leg
• Wrist extensors at the forearm

Legs and Hips

Major muscles of the legs and hips

NAME	JOINTS CROSSED	ORIGIN	INSERTION	ACTION
Gastrocnemius	Ankle and knee	Condyles at the base of the femur	Posterior surface of the calcaneus at the back of the heel	Ankle plantarflexion (strong); Knee flexion (weak)
Soleus	Ankle	Upper ⅔ of the posterior surface of the tibia and fibula	Posterior surface of the calcaneus, at the back of the heel	Ankle plantarflexion
Quadriceps: Rectus femoris	Hip and knee	Anterior, inferior iliac spine of the pelvis	Patella (knee cap) and the patella ligament to the tibial tuberosity	Hip flexion Knee extension
Quadriceps: Vastii: Vastus lateralis Vastus intermedius Vastus medialis	Knee	Lateral, anterior, and medial surface of the femur	Into the patella border	Knee extension
Hamstrings: Short and long biceps femoris (lateral aspect); Semitendinosus and Semimembranosus (medial aspect) (generally work as one muscle)	Hip and knee	Bicep femoris – short head on the posterior femur, on the lower Linea aspera, and the Lateral condyloid ridge. The other heads originate on the Ischial tuberosity of the pelvis.	Biceps femoris inserts onto the head of the fibula and the lateral Condyle of the tibia. Semitendinosus/Semi-membranosus inserts onto the medial Condyle of the tibia	Hip: Extension Knee: Flexion Biceps femoris also actions lateral rotation of the hip and knee. Semitendinosus/Semi-membranosus medially rotate the hip and knee.
Adductor group: Pectineus, Adductor brevis, Adductor longus, Adductor magnus, Gracilis (generally act as one muscle)	Hip (Gracilis also crosses the knee)	Pubis and ischium of the pelvis	Along the medial femur, on the lesser trochanter, linea aspera, and medial condyloid ridge; the Gracilis inserts on the medial superior tibia	Main action is hip adduction
Tensor fasciae latae	Hip	Anterior superior iliac spine	Iliotibial band (ITB)	Hip: abduction, flexion assists medial rotation
Gluteus maximus	Hip	Posterior crest of the ilium, sacrum, and fascia of the lumbar vertebrae	Iliotibial band of the fasciae latae	Hip: extension, lateral rotation
Gluteus medius and minimus (together known as abductors)	Hip	Outer surface of the ilium (both)	Greater trochanter of the femur (both)	Hip: Abduction, lateral rotation (medius), medial rotation (medius, minimus)
Iliopsoas	Hip	Inner surface of the ilium, base of the sacrum; sides of last thoracic and five lumbar vertebrae	Lesser trochanter of the femur	Hip flexion

NEW ANATOMY FOR STRENGTH AND FITNESS TRAINING

NAME	JOINTS CROSSED	ORIGIN	INSERTION	ACTION
Deep lateral rotators of the hip: *Piriformis, Gemellus superior and inferior, Obturator externus and internus, Quadratus femoris (found deep to the gluteus maximus)*	Hip	Anterior sacrum, the posterior ischium and the obturator foramen	Superior and inferior aspects of the greater trochanter	Hip lateral rotation

LEG MUSCLES

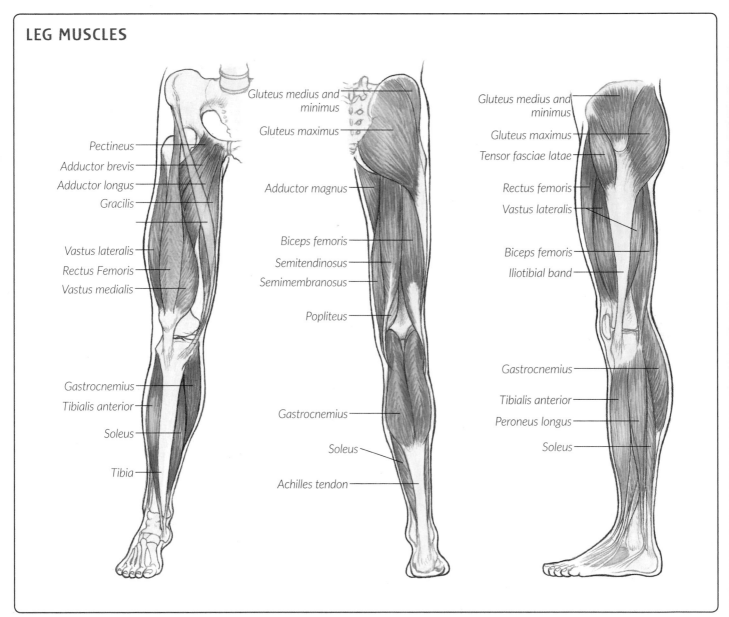

Notes:

Other significant leg muscles, not detailed here for purposes of simplicity, include the Tibialis (both anterior and posterior), the Peroneals, and the Sartorius.

BARBELL LUNGE

Core exercise • Compound/multi-joint
• Push • Closed chain • Barbell
• Beginner to advanced

A progression of the back squat (see page 60) is the lunge, in which one takes a step forward into a squat movement. Many variations are possible, but it is essential that the basic form is correct before proceeding to more advanced versions.

TRAINING TIPS

- Keep the trunk upright and your weight centered between both legs during the exercise.
- Avoid lifting the front heel; keep the front knee from passing over the vertical line of the toes. A common error is too much forward lean from the trunk and pressure on the front knee. Use slow controlled movement.
- Keep the posture aligned and the spine neutral. If the hip flexors are tight, the lumbar alignment will be compromised.
- Keep the chest open, and avoid rounding the shoulders.

ANALYSIS OF MOVEMENT	JOINT 1	JOINT 2
Joints	Hip (front leg)	Knee (front leg)
Joint movement	Down – flexion Up – extension	Down – flexion Up – extension
Mobilizing muscles	Gluteus maximus Hamstring group	Quadricep group

STABILIZING MUSCLES
• Trunk: Abdominal group, Erector spinae, Quadratus lumborum
• Hips: Gluteus medius and minimus, Deep lateral rotators, Adductor group
• Lower leg: Ankle stabilizers, Gastrocnemius

STARTING POSITION

- Stand with your feet shoulder-width apart.
- Support the bar comfortably on the upper Trapezius.
- Step forward with one leg in front of other, so that the front knee is vertically above the front foot. The back leg should be far enough back so that the heel is raised.
- Bend the front leg to lower the body (see opposite).
- Keep your posture aligned and spine neutral.

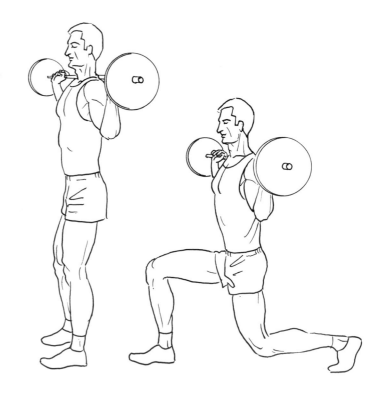

DESCRIPTION

Slowly lower the body by flexing the knee and hip of the front leg to approximately 90° of flexion. The rear knee will almost be touching the ground. Return to the start position and repeat. Swap the front leg and repeat the exercise.

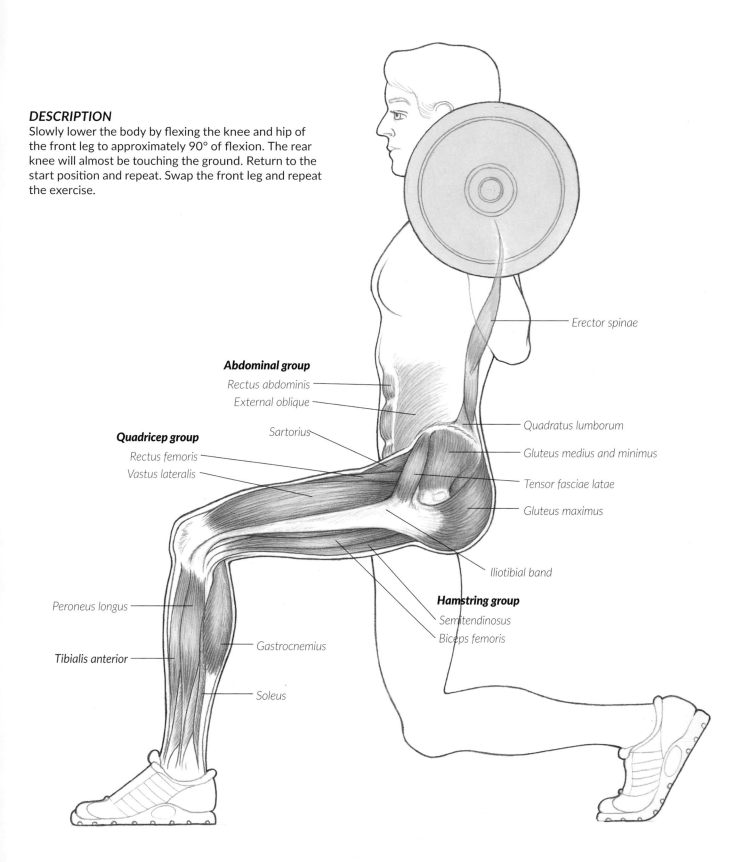

Erector spinae

Abdominal group

Rectus abdominis

External oblique

Quadratus lumborum

Sartorius

Quadricep group

Gluteus medius and minimus

Rectus femoris

Vastus lateralis

Tensor fasciae latae

Gluteus maximus

Iliotibial band

Peroneus longus

Hamstring group

Semitendinosus

Biceps femoris

Tibialis anterior

Gastrocnemius

Soleus

FREESTANDING LATERAL LUNGE

Core exercise • Compound/multi-joint • Push • Close chain • Bodyweight • Beginner to intermediate

This is a variation on the squat and lunge that brings in more activation of the lateral and medial hip and thigh muscles.

TRAINING TIPS

- Keep your posture aligned and your spine neutral.
- Maintain an open chest; avoid rounding your shoulders.
- Keep your knees from passing over the vertical line of your toes; keep your big toe vertically in line with your inside knee.
- Keep your weight directly over your heels to the mid-foot. Avoid lifting your heels.
- If you are unable to maintain lumbar curvature, lower less than 90° at the knees, and start with as little as 45°.
- Inhale on the downwards phase; exhale on the up motion.

STARTING POSITION

- Stand with your feet shoulder-width apart.
- Keep your posture aligned, with a neutral spine.
- Keep your knees soft.

DESCRIPTION

Step one leg sideways, double shoulder-width apart, and slowly lower your body into the squat position, moving your hips back as if sitting into a chair. Lower to approximately 90° of knee flexion, stopping before your upper leg is parallel with the floor. Return, swap legs, and repeat.

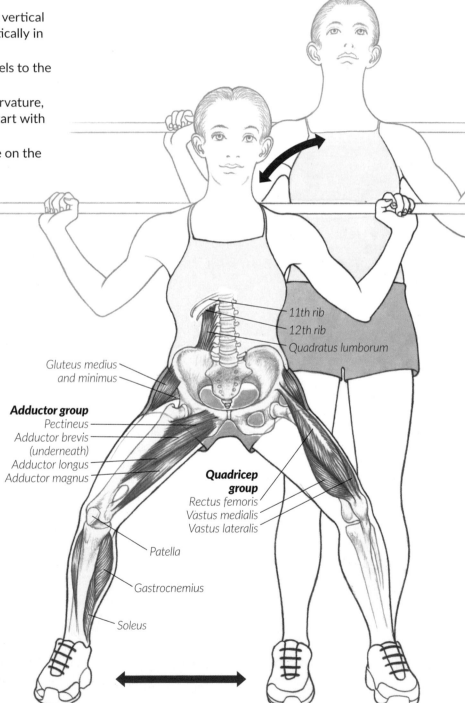

ANALYSIS OF MOVEMENT	JOINT 1	JOINT 2
Joints	Hip	Knee
Joint movement	Down – abduction, then flexion Up – extension, then adduction	Down – flexion Up – extension
Mobilizing muscles	Hip abduction: Gluteus medius and minimus Hip flexion and extension: Gluteus maximus; Hamstring group Hip adduction: Adductor group	Quadricep group

STABILIZING MUSCLES

- Trunk: Abdominal group, Erector spinae, Quadratus lumborum
- Hips: Gluteus medius and minimus, Adductor group (when not mobilizing), Deep lateral rotators

BENCH STEP

Core exercise • Compound/multi-joint • Push • Open chain • Bodyweight • Intermediate to advanced

Using a platform creates an effective workout for the buttock muscles, due to the increased range of hip movement.

DESCRIPTION

With control, step forward up onto the platform. Return to the starting position, controlling the lowering of your body from the leg on the platform.

TRAINING TIPS

- Keep your trunk upright and your weight centered.
- Generate the upward movement by pushing down into the middle and rear of the foot.
- Prevent your front knee from passing over the vertical line of your toes.
- Use a slow, controlled movement. Use a shorter step if you find yourself cheating.
- Keep your posture aligned and your spine neutral.
- Keep your chest open; avoid rounding your shoulders.
- Inhale on the way up.

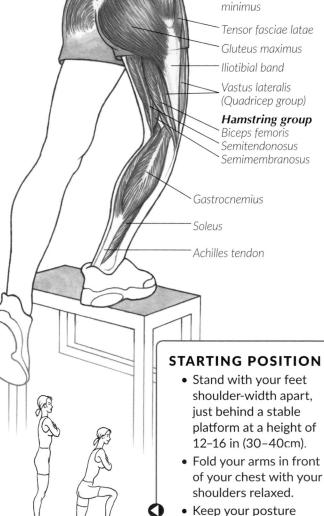

Erector spinae (superficial to Quadratus lumborum)

11th rib
12th rib

Quadratus lumborum (deep)

Gluteus medius and minimus

Tensor fasciae latae

Gluteus maximus

Iliotibial band

Vastus lateralis (Quadricep group)

Hamstring group
Biceps femoris
Semitendonosus
Semimembranosus

Gastrocnemius

Soleus

Achilles tendon

ANALYSIS OF MOVEMENT	JOINT 1	JOINT 2
Joints	Hip (leg stepping up)	Knee (leg stepping up)
Joint movement	Up – flexion, then extension Down – flexion, then extension	Up – flexion, then extension Down – flexion, then extension
Mobilizing muscles	Hip flexion (up): Iliopsoas (Iliopsoas down is passive) Hip extension (up and down): Gluteus maximus, Hamstring group	Knee extension (up) and flexion (down): Quadricep group Knee extension (down): Hamstring group

STABILIZING MUSCLES

- Trunk: Abdominal group, Erector spinae, Quadratus lumborum
- Hips: Gluteus medius and minimus, Deep lateral rotators, Adductor group
- Lower leg: Ankle stabilizers, Gastrocnemius

STARTING POSITION

- Stand with your feet shoulder-width apart, just behind a stable platform at a height of 12–16 in (30–40cm).
- Fold your arms in front of your chest with your shoulders relaxed.
- Keep your posture aligned, and maintain a neutral spine.

FREESTANDING BARBELL PLIÉ SQUATS

Core exercise • Compound/multi-joint • Push • Close chain • Barbell • Intermediate to advanced

There are countless variations possible to the plié squat, which takes it name from the French term meaning "bent." This word refers to the ballet movement of knee bends done with the legs turned out.

DESCRIPTION

Slowly lower your body, moving your hips back as if sitting down on a chair. Lower to approximately 90° of knee flexion, stopping before your upper leg becomes parallel with the floor. Return and repeat.

TRAINING TIPS

- Follow the tips provided for back squats on page 60.

STABILIZING MUSCLES

- Trunk: Abdominal group, Erector spinae, Quadratus lumborum
- Hips: Deep lateral rotators, Gluteus medius and minimus, Adductor group
- Lower legs: Ankle stabilizers, Gastrocnemius

STARTING POSITION

- If using the squat rack, take the bar off the squat rack as described on page 63.
- Stand with your feet double shoulder-width apart and up to 45° outwardly rotated.
- Keep your knees soft.

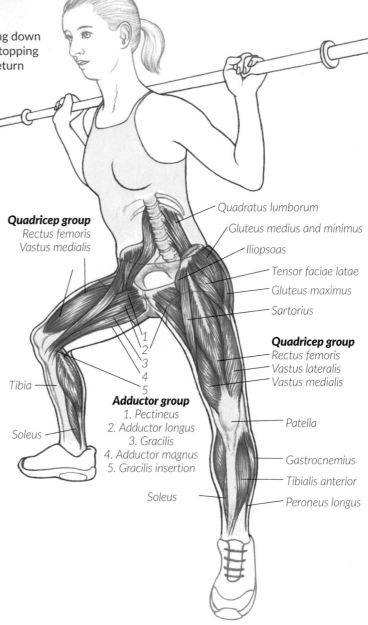

Quadricep group
Rectus femoris
Vastus medialis

Quadratus lumborum
Gluteus medius and minimus
Iliopsoas
Tensor faciae latae
Gluteus maximus
Sartorius

Quadricep group
Rectus femoris
Vastus lateralis
Vastus medialis

Patella

Gastrocnemius
Tibialis anterior
Peroneus longus

Tibia

Soleus

Adductor group
1. Pectineus
2. Adductor longus
3. Gracilis
4. Adductor magnus
5. Gracilis insertion

Soleus

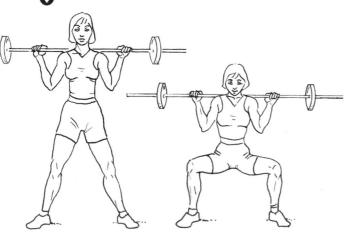

ANALYSIS OF MOVEMENT	JOINT 1	JOINT 2
Joints	Hip	Knee
Joint movement	Down – flexion, abduction Up – extension, adduction	Down – flexion Up – extension
Mobilizing muscles	Gluteus maximus Hamstring group Adductor group	Quadricep group (emphasis is on lateral aspects)

DIFFICULTY   INTERMEDIATE to ADVANCED

SEESAW WITH BALL
Whole body stabilization
• Open chain • Bodyweight • Intermediate
to advanced

This is an unusual and demanding exercise that requires some concentration and stability. It benefits stabilization strength, balance, coordination and proprioceptive skills, and tones the lower back, abdominals, hips, and thighs.

DESCRIPTION
Slowly lean your weight forward by pivoting forward on your hips. At the same time let one extended leg pivot backward as the upper body tilts forward, until you achieve a horizontal line from leg to trunk. Return and repeat, then swap sides.

TRAINING TIPS
- For easier movement, have your standing leg raised by 1–2 in (2–5 cm) on a weight plate or platform.
- Try to keep your chest and shoulders open.
- Maintain posture stabilization throughout.
- Lengthen out in both directions.

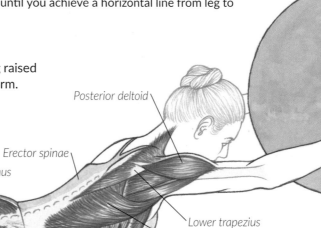

Posterior deltoid

Erector spinae

Gluteus maximus

Lower trapezius

Latissimus dorsi

Serratus anterior

External oblique

Hamstring group
Semimembranosus
Semitendonosus
Biceps femoris

Gluteus medius and minimus

Tensor fasciae latae

Iliotibial band

Vastus lateralis

Gastrocnemius

Tibialis anterior

Peroneus longus

Soleus

ANALYSIS OF MOVEMENT	JOINT 1
Joints	Hips (standing leg)
Joint movement	Forward – flexion Return – extension
Mobilizing muscles	Gluteus maximus Hamstring group

STARTING POSITION
- Stand with your feet shoulder-width apart, with a ball supported between your hands and your arms raised vertically.
- Keep your posture aligned, with your spine neutral.

STABILIZING MUSCLES

The main stabilizers of the trunk are the Abdominal group, Erector spinae, Quadratus lumborum, and muscles of the fixed leg.

- Hips: Gluteus maximus, Hamstring of moving leg
- Upper body: Anterior deltoid, Rotator cuff muscles, Serratus anterior, Rhomboids, Lower trapezius

Plyometrics and Explosive Conditioning

Plyometrics are exercises in which muscles exert maximum force in short intervals of time, with the goal of increasing speed strength (i.e., predominately speed). Plyometrics is a technique that links strength with speed to produce power. "Plyometric training enables a muscle or muscle group to reach its maximum force in the shortest period of time," explains Harvey Newton in the book *Explosive Lifting for Sports*. Whether your sport involves jumping, running, throwing, or lifting, plyometric training can greatly enhance your performance.

In 1964, a Russian scientist named Yuri Verkhoshansky published a system of exercises he called "jump training." It used repetitive jumping in order to increase the speed and explosiveness of Russian track and field athletes. Through the 1960s and 70s, the Soviet Bloc countries dominated the Olympics thanks, in part, to this jump training. American track and field coach Fred Wilt noticed the Russian athletes doing these jumps during their warm-ups. He began to investigate, called them "plyometrics," and took them back to the United States to develop them from there.

Plyometrics include what is known as the stretch-shortening cycle (SSC). This is the loading of a muscle eccentrically followed by rapid concentric muscle contraction. The elastic quality of muscle stores energy in the tissues during the eccentric contraction, just like stretching an elastic band. The subsequent concentric contraction uses the stored energy to contract the muscle more forcibly than the muscle would contract without the prior stretch. The stretch reflex of a muscle is activated when a muscle is lengthened very quickly. The muscle's internal receptors, known as muscle spindles, run the length of the muscle and regulate the rate of change in the length of the muscle. Upon activation of a rapid stretch, the muscle spindles send an afferent nerve impulse to the spinal cord, which then sends an efferent nerve impulse back to the muscle to contract to prevent it over-stretching and tearing. This impulse, along with the release of elastic energy as kinetic energy, produces the increased force production in the SSC.

The stretch reflex, or myotatic reflex, responds to the rate at which the muscle is being stretched and is among the fastest reflexes in the body. The conversion from eccentric to concentric work is known as the amortization phase. This phase lasts just hundredths of a second. The shorter the amortization phase, the greater the force production. Plyometric training enables a shorter amortization phase.

High						
						Depth jumps
					Box drills	
Intensity				Multiple hops and jumps		
			Standing jumps			
		Jumps in place				
Low						

Exercises
Intensity scale for jump exercises, referenced from D. Chu, *Jumping Into Plyometrics*

Number of Foot Contacts by Phase of Training for Jump Training				
	Level			
	Beginner	Intermediate	Advanced	Intensity
Off-season	60–100	100–150	120–200	Low–mod
Pre-season	100–250	150–300	150–450	Mod–high
In-season	Depends on sport			Moderate
Championship season	Recovery only			Mod–high
Adapted from D. Chu, *Jumping Into Plyometrics*				

A WORD ON EXERCISE ANALYSIS IN PLYOMETRICS

With the goal of enhancing learning and understanding, exercise analysis sets out to quantify which joints and muscles are working in a given exercise as well as how they are working (i.e., as stabilizers, mobilizers, concentrically, eccentrically, etc.). The whole-body exercises presented in this section involve most of the muscles of the body in one manner or another.

Additionally, as the exercises consist of several phases, each with its own set of mobilizers and stabilizers, which then transfer emphasis to another set of mobilizers and stabilizers in the next phase, analysis becomes incredibly complex. The flow from one muscle action and function to another is so dynamic that it can be difficult to pinpoint where one starts and one ends. Furthermore, these muscle analyses assume that the exercise is being done correctly by a person of healthy weight, good joint mobility, and postural control and alignment. Any deviation from this can shift emphasis on the joints and muscles actually working in an individual.

Therefore, the muscle analyses in this section should be seen as scientific yet simplified analyses. The human body is an incredible machine, constantly dynamic and far more complex in its function than we are able to represent effectively here.

DIFFICULTY   INTERMEDIATE to ADVANCED

STANDING JUMP AND REACH

Dynamic/plyometric • Compound/multi-joint
Bodyweight • Intermediate to advanced

An ideal warm-up and exercise in itself, the standing jump and reach is an ideal lead-in to more explosive and plyometric work.

DESCRIPTION
Explode upward as if reaching for a target or object.

TRAINING TIPS
- From the half-squat position, drive your feet through the floor and your hips forward.
- Drive your arms forward and up overhead.
- Ensure triple extension of ankles, knees, and hips.

STARTING POSITION
- Stand with your feet shoulder-width apart.
- Drop into a half-squat, arms extended back.

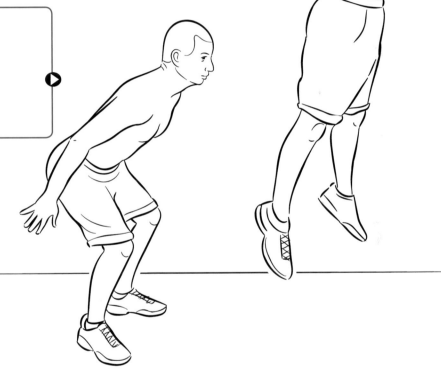

ANALYSIS OF MOVEMENT	Joints	Joint movement	Mobilizing muscles
JOINT 1	Shoulder	Flexion	Anterior deltoid, Pectoralis major (clavicular aspect), Biceps brachii
JOINT 2	Scapula	Upward rotation, abduction (protraction)	Upper and lower trapezius, Pectoralis minor, Serratus anterior
JOINT 3	Spine	Extension	Erector spinae, Multifidus, Rotators, Quadratus lumborum
JOINT 4	Hip	Extension	Gluteus maximus, Gluteus medius, Hamstring group
JOINT 5	Knee	Extension	Quadricep group
JOINT 6	Ankle	Plantarflexion	Gastrocnemius, Soleus, Tibialis posterior, Peroneus longus and brevis

BOX JUMPS

Plyometric exercise • Compound/multi-joint • Close chain • Box • Intermediate to advanced

Box jumps burn calories at a rate of 800 to 1,000 calories per hour, compared to the 200 to 300 calories burned per hour while walking.

DESCRIPTION

Drop into a quarter squat, pushing through the soles of both feet, and immediately rebound and accelerate, jumping onto the box. As you land in a squat, extend your hips and knees fully to stand in an upright position. Pause. Return and repeat. Land in the same position as you took off.

BOX JUMP ESSENTIALS

The popularity of high-intensity strength and conditioning programs, especially CrossFit, has brought box jumping into the functional multimode training environment. In order to perform box jumps, you need a special box. Often known as "plyo boxes," these boxes usually range in height from 12–24 in (30–60cm), with 24 in (60cm) being the preferred CrossFit standard. Beginners are likely to start on 12-in (30-cm) boxes. Though boxes can be homemade, they should have slip-proof surfaces, stable bases, and be able to take up to 250 lbs (113kg) of landing weight. In choosing a box of the correct height, a good rule of thumb is to pick a box that you can jump onto and get both feet completely onto the box. If you land in an extremely deep squat, it's likely your box is too high. If you cannot land full foot and quietly (like a cat), it's also likely too high. Your age, weight, injury history, flexibility, and plyometric ability, not to mention training goals, are all valid considerations in choosing both box height and what type of box jump to begin training with.

Box jumping is an explosive exercise and should be programmed before heavy lifting and after a warm-up; it is better used in these ways than as a prolonged exercise in itself. It can help explosive strength, speed agility, coordination, accuracy, and balance. That said, box jumps are not for everyone, and they should only be brought into a program one basic foundational flexibility and postural strength have been secured.

The box jump has significantly less impact stress on the joints than, for example, standing vertical jumps (see page 93), especially when the eccentric return phase is kept low impact. Thus, box jumps can be trained more frequently compared to other higher-impact variations. The box jump also has less shear stress and compressive stress at the knee.

For the average person not training for peak athletic performance, it is recommended to start with box jumps for 2–3 sets of 3–5 reps. High volume isn't important; high performance with good quality form is.

TRAINING TIPS

GENERAL

- This cannot be stressed enough: quality is more important than quantity, without compromise to training intensity. Full hip extension on your jump and building sound landing mechanics is the most important thing, not height.
- Full hip extension helps improve the foundation of other power lifts and athletic movements.
- Throughout, knees are neutral, rather than in valgus or varus (i.e., knock-kneed or bowlegged). As a rule, keep the medial kneecap vertically in line with the big toe.
- The focus is on jumping up and down, not long jumping forward.

TAKEOFF

- Brace and maintain the arch of the lumbar spine.
- Focus and concentrate on your intended landing spot while your head and eyes are aimed just above the horizon.
- As you drop into the squat, prior to jumping, imagine loading your Hamstrings and glutes and recoiling upward as you jump up.
- Once off the ground, tuck your knees up in order to clear the box and land on top.
- Use your arms to aid your momentum, but drive your power from your lower body.

STABILIZING MUSCLES

Dynamic stabilization is key in controlling the momentum and explosive acceleration in this exercise.

- Lower and Mid trapezius, Levator scapula, Rhomboids, and Serratus anterior at the shoulder blades
- Rotator cuff group, Deltoids, and arm muscles
- Abdominal group, Erector spinae, and Quadratus lumborum at the trunk
- Gluteus medius and minimus, Deep lateral rotators, and the Adductor group at the hips
- Ankle stabilizers, Tibialis anterior, and Gastrocnemius in the lower leg

STARTING POSITION

- Stand with feet hip to shoulder distance apart, at a comfortable distance from the box.
- Keep your posture aligned, with a neutral spine.

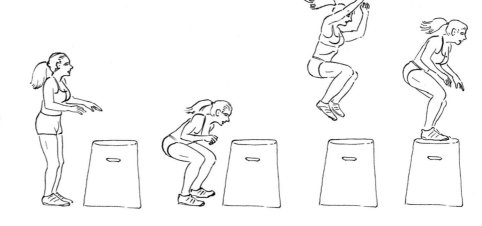

LANDING

- Land on your full feet, flat.
- Try to land quietly. If you find you are struggling with the landing, it's a good sign to lower the box height.
- Eyes and chest are up. Avoid dropping the head and rounding the shoulders.

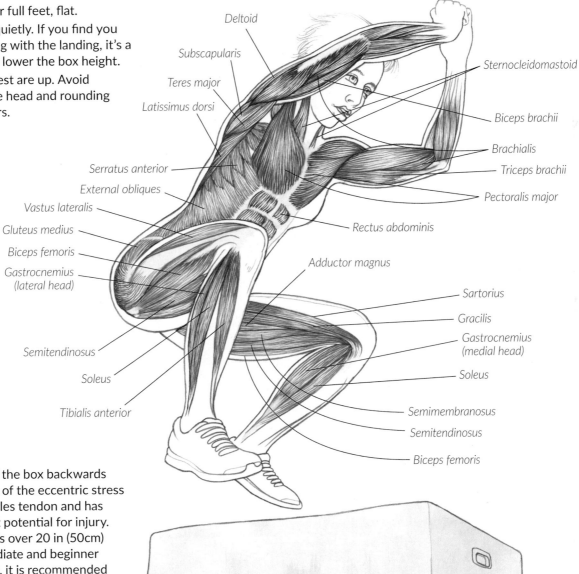

Deltoid

Subscapularis

Teres major

Latissimus dorsi

Serratus anterior

External obliques

Vastus lateralis

Gluteus medius

Biceps femoris

Gastrocnemius (lateral head)

Semitendinosus

Soleus

Tibialis anterior

Sternocleidomastoid

Biceps brachii

Brachialis

Triceps brachii

Pectoralis major

Rectus abdominis

Adductor magnus

Sartorius

Gracilis

Gastrocnemius (medial head)

Soleus

Semimembranosus

Semitendinosus

Biceps femoris

24" (60cm) box

RETURN

- Jumping off the box backwards places most of the eccentric stress on the Achilles tendon and has the greatest potential for injury. If your box is over 20 in (50cm) for intermediate and beginner nonathletes, it is recommended that you step backwards in the return phase.
- Re-bend when landing to absorb your jump back down.

DIFFICULTY · **INTERMEDIATE to ADVANCED**

WALL BALLS

Compound/multi-joint • Close chain • Medicine ball • Intermediate to advanced

Wall balls can help to build the foundation of the 9 CrossFit movements as well as a range of plyometric and explosive sports-specific movements.

DESCRIPTION

From the squat position, accelerate upward, extending at the hips and knees. Let the momentum transfer to the ball, throwing it upward against the wall to reach the target. In sync with your squat return, catch the ball and smoothly descend to the squat bottom position. Flow into the next repetition.

MEDICINE BALL ESSENTIALS

The medicine ball is one of the oldest and most versatile exercise tools to have made its way into mainstream, modern, multimode functional training. As far back as 3,000 years ago, Persian wrestlers were depicted training with sand-filled bladders. In 1876, Robert J. Roberts gave the medicine ball its modern name, derived from a similar American Indian ball called a "medicine bag."

Generally, medicine balls nowadays have a softer, more pillowy feel than the original versions. They have some degree of bounce. They are generally 14 in (36 cm) in diameter and are available from 2 to 28 lbs (1 to 12kg). For most beginners, 4 to 8 lbs (2 to 4kg) is a good starting ball weight. The rule of thumb in choosing the right medicine ball for you is to choose a ball just heavy enough to provide resistance, but not so heavy as to alter the proper form and speed of the selected movement.

The medicine ball is an invaluable tool and has wide potential for application to help build strength and explosive power through high-intensity training. A wide range of sporting codes and athletes as well as exercise types (including CrossFit) use medicine balls for explosive, plyometric, and power training as well as sport-specific conditioning.

As with other exercises, increasing with higher volume sets and greater speed of movement and explosiveness with reciprocating lower ball weight will train the speed, endurance, and explosive power response in an individual. Lower weight is also more suited to sport-specific movement pattern development. Heavier ball weight with slower, lower volume sets will increase the emphasis on weight training effect for strength gains.

Proficiency in the air squat (see page 58) should be achieved before advancing to wall balls, as well as ensuring adequate flexibility and neuromuscular control.

TRAINING TIPS

- Standing too far from the wall will limit effectiveness and increase strain; too close and you'll not get proper extension. To find the correct distance, stand with the ball in hand, arms fully straightened in front of you. Where the ball touches the wall is the right distance.
- Keep the ball closer to the chest and through the throw. This keeps the resistance arm (lever) short. That said, keep your arms up and your concentration on the ball. It's heavy—face smashes are possible.
- Heels remain down until hips and knees fully extend, then naturally transition into jump phase. For a scaled-back version, keep heels flat on the ground.
- Maintain a graceful pace throughout the movement, rather than stoping and starting. When the ball descends, absorb it into your body rather than catching

STARTING POSITION

- Descend into the squat position.
- With you heels flat, keep your knees vertically in line with the toes and feet shoulder distance apart.
- Keep your posture aligned, with a neutral spine, eyes looking slightly above horizon. Look at your target.
- Hold the ball to your chest, with elbows under the ball and forward.
- You can go into a deep knee squat, provided you have no joint or injury limitations and that you are able to maintain proper form.

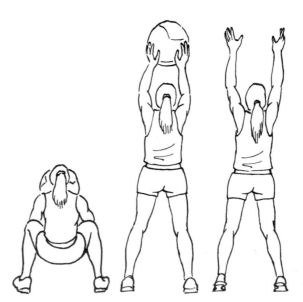

ANALYSIS OF MOVEMENT

LOWER BODY	JOINT 1	JOINT 2	JOINT 3
Joints	Ankle	Knee	Hip
Joint movement	Up – plantarflexion	Up – extension	Up – extension
Mobilizing muscles	Gastrocnemius Soleus	Quadricep group	Gluteus maximus Hamstring group
UPPER BODY	**JOINT 4**	**JOINT 5**	**JOINT 6**
Joints	Elbow	Shoulder	Scapulothoracic
Joint movement	Up – extension	Up – flexion, abduction, lateral rotation	Up – upward rotation
Mobilizing muscles	Triceps brachii Anconeus	Deltoid Supraspinatus Infraspinatus Teres minor Pectoralis major (clavicular aspect)	Upper trapezius Levator scapula Serratus anterior

Note: *For the purpose of simplicity, only the active phase has been detailed (i.e., the up phase of the exercise).*

it. Keep the elbows high. Do not rest the elbows on the knees.

- Brace and maintain the arch of the lumbar spine.
- Don't drop the head—maintain eye level just above horizontal with a neutral cervical spine.
- Keep chest open, avoiding rounding the shoulders.
- Keep your weight directly over the heel to mid-foot.
- If there are joint or injury limitations at the knee, only go down to 90° (i.e., keep your hips above the knees in the squat).
- If you can do the deep knee version, try practicing with another ball placed on the floor behind you that you "sit" on during each rep. Don't actually sit on the ball—just touch it.

STABILIZING MUSCLES

Dynamic stabilization is key in controlling the momentum and explosive acceleration in this exercise.

- Lower and Mid trapezius, Levator scapula, Rhomboids, and Serratus anterior at the shoulder blades
- Rotator cuff group, Deltoids, and arm muscles
- Abdominal group, Erector spinae, and Quadratus lumborum at the trunk
- Gluteus medius and minimus, Deep lateral rotators, and the Adductor group at the hips
- Ankle stabilizers, Tibialis anterior, and Gastrocnemius in the lower leg

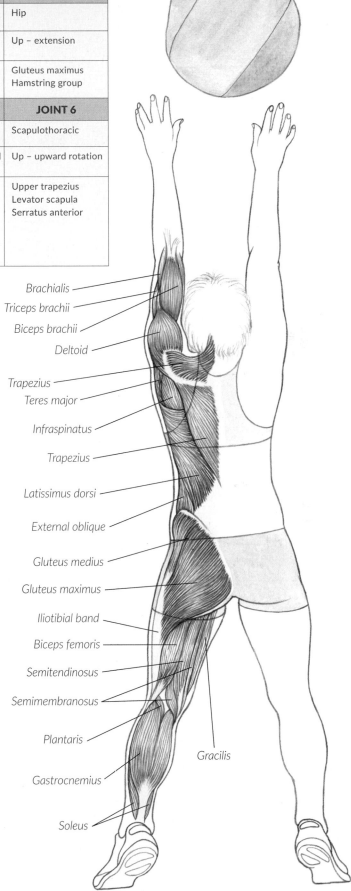

Brachialis
Triceps brachii
Biceps brachii
Deltoid
Trapezius
Teres major
Infraspinatus
Trapezius
Latissimus dorsi
External oblique
Gluteus medius
Gluteus maximus
Iliotibial band
Biceps femoris
Semitendinosus
Semimembranosus
Plantaris
Gracilis
Gastrocnemius
Soleus

DIFFICULTY **INTERMEDIATE to ADVANCED**

4-POINT BURPEE

Compound/multi-joint • Close chain • Bodyweight • Intermediate to advanced

On May 17, 2014, Cameron Dorn made two burpee world records: 5,657 burpees performed in 12 hours, and 10,105 in 24 hours.

DESCRIPTION

THE ORIGINAL 4-POINT BURPEE:

- From standing, squat down and place both hands on the floor in front of you.
- Jump feet back into plank position.
- Jump feet forward back into 2nd position (i.e., squat).
- Return to standing.

ADVANCED CROSSFIT 6-POINT VERSION:

- From standing, squat down and place both hands on the floor in front of you.
- Jump feet back into plank position.
- Drop to a push-up; chest should touch the floor.
- Return to plank.
- Jump feet forward back into 2nd position.
- Transition into an explosive upward jump up, reaching arms straight overhead. Land into quarter squat and return to standing.

BURPEE ESSENTIALS

The burpee was developed by American physiologist Royal Huddleston Burpee, who developed the exercise at the YMCA Bronx in 1939 as part of his PhD thesis. Burpee was looking for a quick and simple way to assess fitness in ordinary individuals. In his protocol, the burpee was a simple 4-point movement. In the 70 years since the burpee's birth, thanks to the popularity of high-intensity strength and conditioning programs, many variations of the original 4-point exercise have been developed and evolved, including the standard 6-point CrossFit burpee, which contains a push-up in the middle and a plyometric jump at the end.

Burpees have been called the complete exercise for good reason; consider that the 4-point burpee involves a squat, a jump, a plank, another jump, and a squat. As a multi-joint compound exercise, it overloads strength, endurance, and flexibility, not to mention developing agility, coordination, power, and balance.

Burpees should be regarded as an advanced exercise. Proficiency in the air squat (see page 58), the plank (see page 48), and the push-up (see page 102) should be achieved before advancing to burpees, as well as ensuring adequate flexibility and neuromuscular control.

ANALYSIS OF MOVEMENT

The burpee is one of the most complete exercises in terms of the use of muscular mobilizers and stabilizers. The 4-point burpee can be divided into 4 main phases (see the description). The complex analysis of muscle use is almost mindboggling. In short:

In Phase 1, the hips and knees flex. As gravity is largely acting on the body here, it is the Quadricep at the knees, the Hamstrings and Gluteus maximus at the hip, and the Gastrocnemius and Soleus at the ankle that contract eccentrically (i.e., lengthen under tension).

In Phase 2, as the weight of the upper body transitions into the hands, the upper body muscles largely stabilize the posture. The postural load increases as the legs kick back, lengthening the body into the plank position. The Erector spinae, Abdominals, and all deep muscles of the trunk, as well as of the legs, hips, arms, and shoulders, dynamically stabilize and align the body in its now prone position (facing down). To kick the legs back into the plank, the Gluteus and Hamstrings at the hip and the Quadriceps at the knees extend these joints by now contracting concentrically.

Phase 3 sees concentric contraction of the Rectus femoris (long head of the Quadriceps) and Iliopsoas, flexing the hips, with supplementary contraction of the Gastrocnemius and Hamstrings flexing the knees, to land back in the squat. The acceleration of the feet forward is activated by rapid plantarflexion of the ankle by the calf muscles, not to mention the countless lower leg muscles facilitating toe movements. Upper body, trunk, and hip muscles continue to stabilize the posture.

In Phase 4, returning to the standing position movement is largely through extension of the hip by concentric contraction of the Gluteus maximus and Hamstrings. At the knee the Hamstrings contract concentrically, the calf muscles at the ankle. Stabilization load reduces as the body moves upright, offering less resistance to gravity, though stabilization is still active.

This summary does not adequately convey the minutiae of muscles mobilizing and stabilizing the body. If the CrossFit version is followed, additional muscles are involved in mobilizing, and explosive mobilization drives the plyometric jump added at the end. For these muscles analyses, see the plank (page 48), the push-up (page 102), and the standing jump and reach (page 93).

STARTING POSITION

- Stand with your feet shoulder-width apart.
- With heels flat, keep your knees vertically in line with your toes.
- Keep your feet shoulder distance apart.
- Keep your posture aligned and your spine neutral.

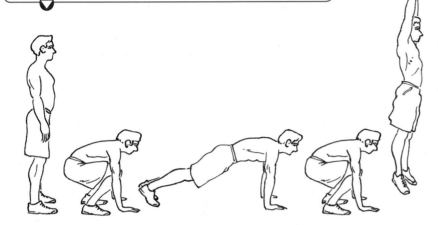

TRAINING TIPS

GENERAL

- This cannot be stressed enough: quality is more important than quantity, without compromise to training intensity.
- Go slow and steady in pace, rather than stop and start, which tends to result in low-quality motor control. Pace your breathing, too. Lack of oxygen will lead to premature failure.
- Easier versions include moving the legs back and forward one at a time rather than jumping.

COMMON ERRORS

- If the Hamstrings are tight, one tends to bend more at the hips and less at the knees, increasing stress on the lower back and reducing the effectiveness of the exercise. To protect the lower back, it is highly recommended to squat with feet shoulder-width apart, and hands inside the feet, while squatting down with the legs, not the back.
- Avoid coming out of the plank by lifting the back (i.e., going into a downward dog). Rather, maintain spinal stabilization and use the legs to jump forward.
- Avoid sagging in the plank position. Keep the chest open, avoiding rounding the shoulders.
- If form is compromised, do fewer 4-point burpees, and improve ability and form in the air squat and plank, as well as in Hamstring and other hip extensors flexibility.

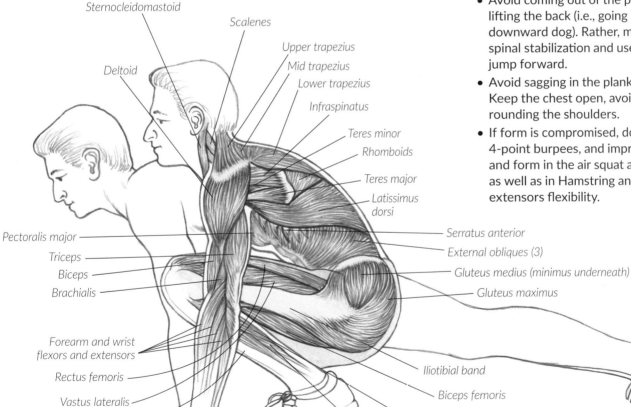

Sternocleidomastoid
Scalenes
Upper trapezius
Mid trapezius
Lower trapezius
Infraspinatus
Teres minor
Rhomboids
Teres major
Latissimus dorsi
Deltoid
Pectoralis major
Triceps
Biceps
Brachialis
Forearm and wrist flexors and extensors
Rectus femoris
Vastus lateralis
Tibialis anterior
Serratus anterior
External obliques (3)
Gluteus medius (minimus underneath)
Gluteus maximus
Iliotibial band
Biceps femoris
Gastrocnemius
Soleus

Chest

A simple tip: if you are looking for a fuller bust, proper upper body posture will enhance this. Conversely, rounding your shoulders will make your chest look flatter. Include a balance of mid- and upper-back exercises and some time on a rowing machine to enhance the strength of the postural muscles that keep the chest open and the shoulders relaxed.

The Serratus anterior acts as a dynamic stabilizer by depressing the shoulder blades and keeping them flat against the back. "Hanging" from the shoulder blades while doing chest exercises such as push-ups is a sign of a weak/inactive Serratus anterior and should be avoided. Instead, aim to depress and widen the shoulder blades against your back, thereby activating the Serratus anterior and Lower trapezius. This stabilization principle applies to all chest exercises.

Muscles involved in chest exercises

NAME	JOINTS CROSSED	ORIGIN	INSERTION	ACTION
Pectoralis major	Shoulder	• Clavicular (upper portion)—medial half of the anterior surface of the clavicle • Sternal (mid-portion) and abdominal (lower) portion • Anterior surface of the costal cartilages of the first 6 ribs and the adjoining portion of the sternum	Flat tendon of the intertubercular groove of the humerus	**Shoulder:** • adduction • horizontal adduction • internal rotation • flexion
Pectoralis minor	Scapula to ribs	Anterior surface of the 3rd to the 5th ribs	Coracoid process of the scapula	**Scapula:** • abduction (protraction) • downward rotation • depression
Anterior deltoid	Shoulder	Anterior lateral third of the clavicle	Lateral side of the humerus	**Shoulder:** • flexion • horizontal flexion • medial rotation
Triceps brachii	Shoulder and elbow	Scapula and upper posterior humerus	The olecranon process of the ulna	Elbow extension
Serratus anterior	Shoulder	Upper 9 ribs at the side of the chest	Anterior aspect of the entire medial border of the scapula	**Scapula:** • abduction (protraction) • upward rotation
Coracobrachialis	Shoulder	Coracoid process of the scapula	Middle medial border of humeral shaft	**Shoulder:** • horizontal adduction
Anconeus	Elbow	Posterior lateral condyle of the humerus	Posterior surface of the olecranon process of the ulna	Elbow extension (works with the triceps)

Note:

The Triceps brachii is detailed under Arms (see page 130).

CHEST MUSCLES

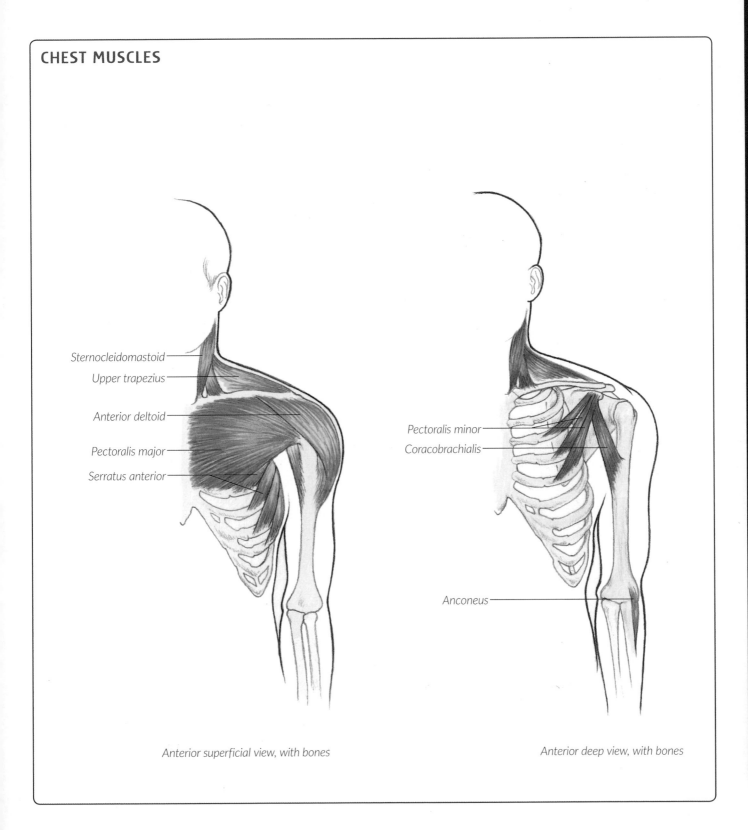

Sternocleidomastoid

Upper trapezius

Anterior deltoid

Pectoralis major

Serratus anterior

Pectoralis minor

Coracobrachialis

Anconeus

Anterior superficial view, with bones

Anterior deep view, with bones

DIFFICULTY — BEGINNER to ADVANCED

PUSH-UPS

Core exercise • Compound/ multi-joint
• Push • Close chain • Bodyweight
• Functional • Beginner to advanced

Paddy Doyle, of the UK, currently holds the Guinness World Record for the most push-ups done in one year (1988–89): a phenomenal 1,500,230!

DESCRIPTION

Maintaining posture, lower the body to the floor by bending the elbows. Return by pushing the body up until the arms are straight and the elbows are extended. Repeat.

TRAINING TIPS

- Use slow, controlled movement.
- Maintain spinal alignment.
- Avoid compensating with momentum.

STABILIZING MUSCLES

- A push-up has a stronger stabilization emphasis than in the bench press (see page 106).
- Shoulder blades: Serratus anterior, Pectoralis minor, Rhomboids, Lower trapezius
- Shoulder joint: Rotator cuff muscles, Biceps brachii
- Trunk stabilization: Abdominal, Gluteal and Quadricep group, Quadratus lumborum, Latissimus dorsi

STARTING POSITION

- Begin by lying prone.
- Raise up your body, supporting it on your hands and toes.
- Extend your arms, keeping them slightly wider than shoulder-width at upper chest level.
- Keep your posture aligned.

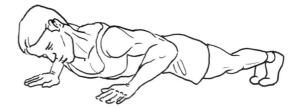

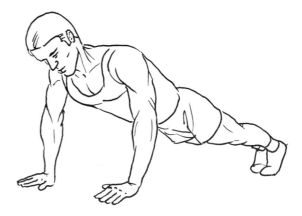

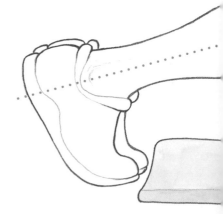

ANALYSIS OF MOVEMENT	JOINT 1	JOINT 2	JOINT 3
Joints	Elbow	Shoulder	Scapulothoracic
Joint movement	Up – extension Down – flexion	Up – horizontal adduction, flexion Down – horizontal abduction, extension	Up – partial upward rotation, abduction Down – partial downward rotation, adduction
Mobilizing muscles	Triceps brachii Anconeus	Pectoralis major, emphasis on the sternal and clavicular aspect Coracobrachialis Anterior deltoid	Serratus anterior

PROGRESSING PUSH-UPS

Push-ups can be progressed (i.e., made harder) in countless ways. Doing push-ups using balls or modifying with kettlebells, dumbbells, or alternate hand, arm, leg, and foot positions are just a few of the typical changes that can be made. Increasing repetitions, sets, and speed, reducing rest periods, and adding declines (feet higher than shoulders) progress the overload of push-ups, too. In CrossFit, an inverted wall push-up (i.e., a handstand push-up) is an advanced and coveted achievement. As always, do not progress the exercise until you can do standard push-ups with good form while maintaining proper postural stabilization and alignment.

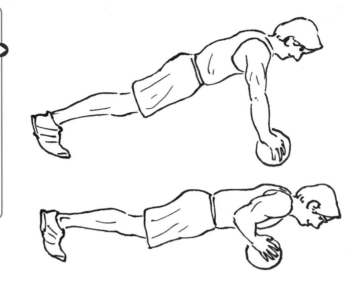

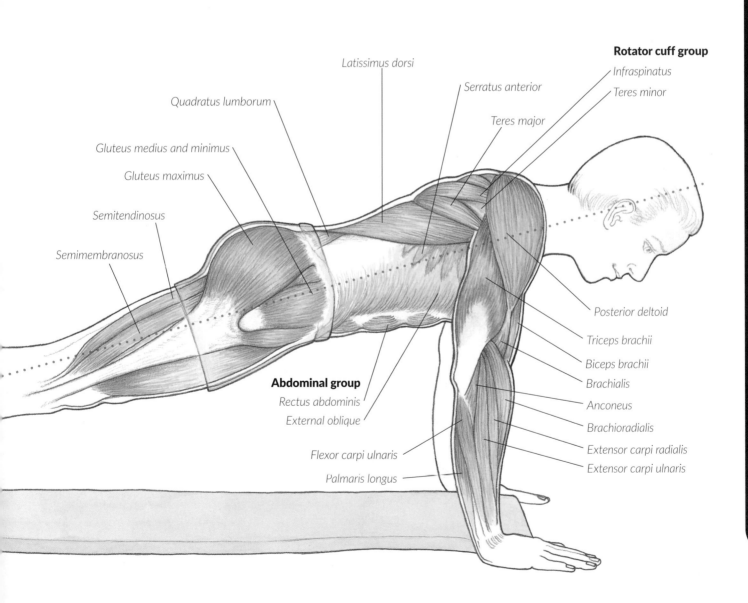

Latissimus dorsi

Serratus anterior

Rotator cuff group

Infraspinatus

Teres minor

Teres major

Quadratus lumborum

Gluteus medius and minimus

Gluteus maximus

Semitendinosus

Semimembranosus

Posterior deltoid

Triceps brachii

Biceps brachii

Brachialis

Anconeus

Brachioradialis

Extensor carpi radialis

Extensor carpi ulnaris

Abdominal group

Rectus abdominis

External oblique

Flexor carpi ulnaris

Palmaris longus

DIFFICULTY   **BEGINNER to ADVANCED**

BODYWEIGHT MODIFIED PUSH-UPS

Core exercise • Compound/multi-joint • Push
• Close chain • Bodyweight • Functional • Beginner
to advanced

Renata Hamplová from the Czech Republic holds the women's world record for the most push-ups over 3 and over 10 minutes, both set in 1995. She managed to do 190 and 426 push-ups, respectively.

DESCRIPTION

Maintaining your postural alignment, lower your body to the floor by bending at the elbows. Return by pushing up until your arms are straight. Repeat.

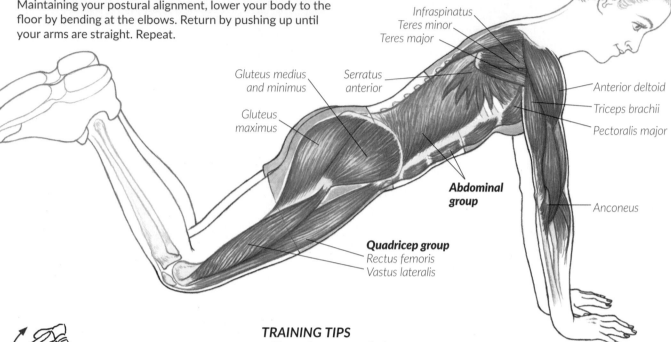

Infraspinatus
Teres minor
Teres major
Gluteus medius and minimus
Serratus anterior
Anterior deltoid
Triceps brachii
Pectoralis major
Gluteus maximus
Abdominal group
Anconeus
Quadricep group
Rectus femoris
Vastus lateralis

TRAINING TIPS

• Use a slow, controlled movement.
• Maintain alignment, keeping your ears, shoulders, hips, and knees in line.
• Avoid compensating with momentum.
• Avoid "hanging" from your shoulder blades. Aim to depress and widen your shoulder blades by keeping them flat against your back.

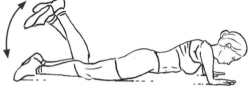

STARTING POSITION

• Lie in a prone position.
• Raise up your body, supported on your hands and knees.
• Extend your arms slightly wider than shoulder-width apart, at upper chest level.
• Keep your posture aligned.

STABILIZING MUSCLES

• Shoulder blades: Serratus anterior, Pectoralis minor, Rhomboids, Lower trapezius
• Shoulder joints: Rotator cuff muscles, Biceps brachii
• Trunk stabilization: Abdominal, Gluteal and Quadricep group, Quadratus lumborum, Latissimus dorsi

ANALYSIS OF MOVEMENT	JOINT 1	JOINT 2	JOINT 3
Joints	Elbow	Shoulder	Scapulothoracic
Joint movement	Up – extension Down – flexion	Up – horizontal adduction, flexion Down – horizontal abduction, extension	Up – partial upwards rotation, abduction (protraction) Down – partial downwards rotation, adduction (retraction)
Mobilizing muscles	Triceps brachii Anconeus	Pectoralis major, emphasis on the sternal and clavicular aspects Coracobrachialis Anterior deltoid	Serratus anterior

DIFFICULTY | **BEGINNER to ADVANCED**

DUMBBELL BENCH PRESS

Core exercise • Compound/multi-joint
• Push • Open chain • Dumbbell
• Beginner to advanced

A greater range of motion is possible here than in the barbell bench press (see page 106), allowing you to work your muscles through a greater range of motion. More stabilization is needed, as the weights need to be controlled independently.

DESCRIPTION

Bending the elbows, lower the dumbbells in line with the upper chest. Return by pressing until the arms are extended. Repeat.

TRAINING TIPS

- Establish good form before increasing weight.
- Avoid momentum; use slow, controlled motion.
- On the up motion, do not bring the dumbbells together completely; keep them about 6 in (15cm) apart.
- Breathe out when raising the dumbbells.

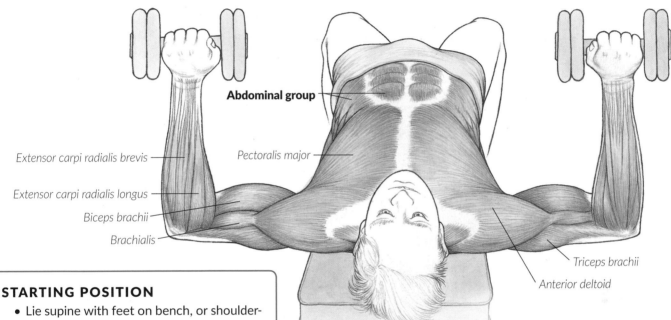

Abdominal group

Extensor carpi radialis brevis

Extensor carpi radialis longus

Biceps brachii

Brachialis

Pectoralis major

Triceps brachii

Anterior deltoid

STARTING POSITION

- Lie supine with feet on bench, or shoulder-width on ground for stability. Keep spine aligned.
- Lift dumbbells to knees, using momentum.
- Dumbbells are at upper chest level, supported vertically above elbows.

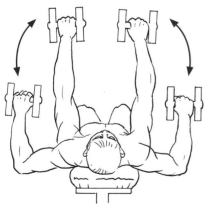

STABILIZING MUSCLES

- Shoulder blades: Serratus anterior, Pectoralis minor, Rhomboids, Lower trapezius
- Shoulder joint: Rotator cuff muscles, Biceps brachii
- Mild trunk stabilization: Abdominal and Gluteal group, Latissimus dorsi

ANALYSIS OF MOVEMENT	JOINT 1	JOINT 2	JOINT 3
Joints	Elbow	Shoulder	Scapulothoracic
Joint movement	Up – extension Down – flexion	Up – horizontal adduction, flexion Down – horizontal abduction, extension	Up – partial upward rotation, abduction Down – partial downward rotation, adduction
Mobilizing muscles	Triceps brachii	Pectoralis major, emphasis on the sternal and clavicular aspect Coracobrachialis Anterior deltoid	Serratus anterior

BARBELL BENCH PRESS

Core exercise • Compound/multi-joint
• Push • Open chain • Barbell
• Intermediate to advanced

In the Strongest Man in the World competition, Anthony Clark, from the Philippines, bench pressed a massive 800 lbs (363kg). Since he weighs 350 lbs (159kg), that's nearly two and a half times his own bodyweight!

DESCRIPTION

Dismount the bar from the rack. Bending the elbows, lower the bar in line with the upper chest. Return by pressing upwards until arms are extended. Repeat.

TRAINING TIPS

- Achieve good form before increasing weight.
- Avoid momentum; use slow, controlled motion.
- Breathe out when raising the bar.

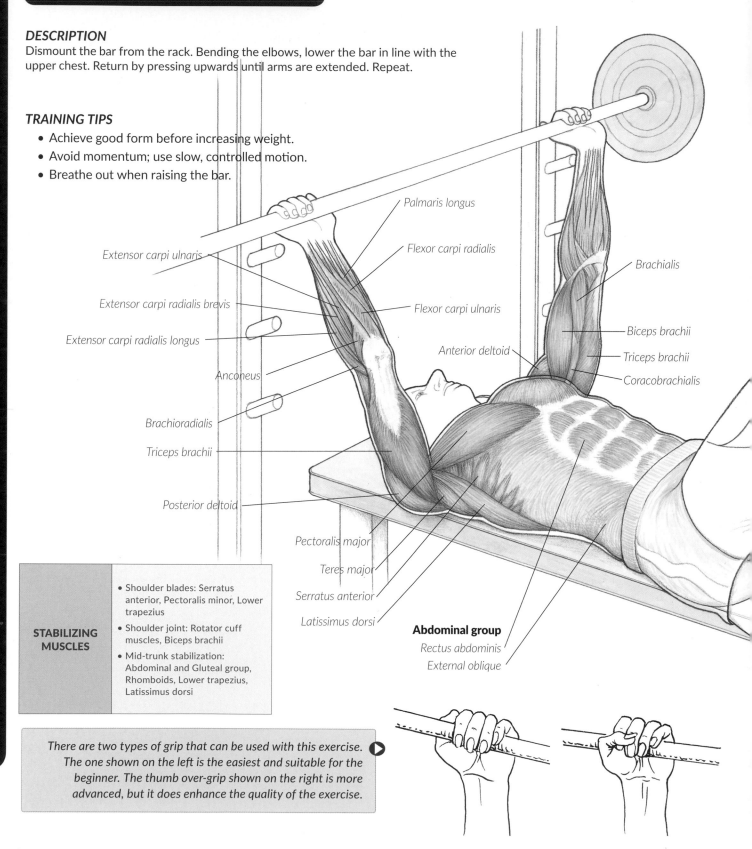

Palmaris longus

Flexor carpi radialis

Extensor carpi ulnaris

Extensor carpi radialis brevis

Flexor carpi ulnaris

Brachialis

Extensor carpi radialis longus

Anterior deltoid

Biceps brachii

Triceps brachii

Anconeus

Coracobrachialis

Brachioradialis

Triceps brachii

Posterior deltoid

Pectoralis major

Teres major

Serratus anterior

Latissimus dorsi

Abdominal group

Rectus abdominis

External oblique

STABILIZING MUSCLES	• Shoulder blades: Serratus anterior, Pectoralis minor, Lower trapezius • Shoulder joint: Rotator cuff muscles, Biceps brachii • Mid-trunk stabilization: Abdominal and Gluteal group, Rhomboids, Lower trapezius, Latissimus dorsi

There are two types of grip that can be used with this exercise. The one shown on the left is the easiest and suitable for the beginner. The thumb over-grip shown on the right is more advanced, but it does enhance the quality of the exercise.

ANALYSIS OF MOVEMENT	JOINT 1	JOINT 2	JOINT 3
Joints	Elbow	Shoulder	Scapulothoracic
Joint movement	Up – extension Down – flexion	Up – horizontal adduction, flexion Down – horizontal abduction, extension	Up – partial upward rotation, abduction Down – partial downward rotation, adduction
Mobilizing muscles	Triceps brachii Anconeus	Pectoralis major, emphasis on the sternal and clavicular aspect Coracobrachialis Anterior deltoid	Serratus anterior

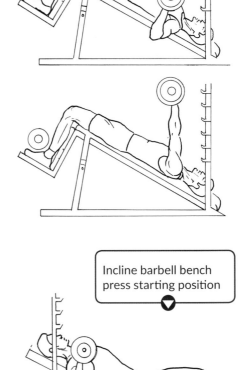

Decline barbell bench press starting position

STARTING POSITION

- Begin by lying supine.
- Use a medium grip (slightly wider than shoulder-width).
- Keep your spine aligned (if appropriate, raise feet onto the bench to reduce arching in the lower back).

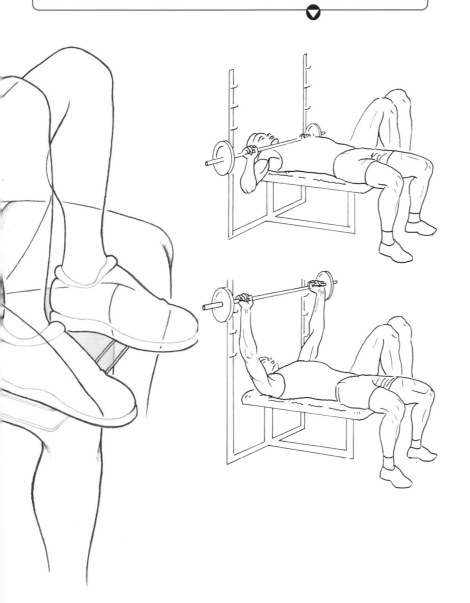

Incline barbell bench press starting position

DIFFICULTY **BEGINNER to ADVANCED**

DUMBBELL FLAT BENCH FLYES

*Auxiliary exercise • Isolation/single joint • Push
• Open chain • Dumbbell • Beginner to advanced*

The dumbbells used in this exercise originated in India in the 11th century, when stone weights known as *nals* were used in "gyms" by those performing strength-training exercises.

DESCRIPTION
Lower the dumbbells to your sides until your chest muscles are stretched. Return and repeat.

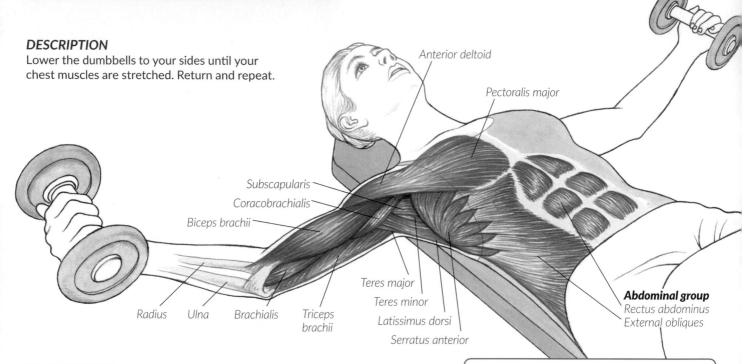

- Anterior deltoid
- Pectoralis major
- Subscapularis
- Coracobrachialis
- Biceps brachii
- Radius
- Ulna
- Brachialis
- Triceps brachii
- Teres major
- Teres minor
- Latissimus dorsi
- Serratus anterior
- **Abdominal group**
  Rectus abdominus
  External obliques

TRAINING TIPS
- Avoid overextending your elbows and tensing your shoulders. Keep your elbows extended with a 10° bend.
- Establish good form before increasing the weight.
- Avoid momentum.
- Breathe out when raising the dumbbells.

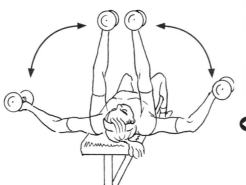

STARTING POSITION
- Lift the dumbbells to your knees, then, while lying back, use momentum to lift them to the starting position.
- Lie supine with your feet on a bench or shoulder-width apart on the ground for stability.
- Start with your arms extended.
- Keep your spine aligned with your feet raised on the bench.

STABILIZING MUSCLES
• Shoulder blades: Serratus anterior, Pectoralis minor, Rhomboids, Lower trapezius
• Shoulder joints: Rotator cuff muscles, Biceps brachii
• Elbow joints: Triceps brachii, Brachialis
• Wrists: Wrist flexors
• Mild trunk stabilization: Abdominal and Gluteal group, Latissimus dorsi

ANALYSIS OF MOVEMENT	JOINT 1	JOINT 2
Joints	Shoulder	Scapulothoracic
Joint movement	Up – horizontal adduction Down – horizontal abduction	Inward – partial abduction (protraction) Return – partial adduction (retraction)
Mobilizing muscles	Pectoralis major, emphasis on the sternal and clavicular aspect Coracobrachialis Anterior deltoid Biceps brachii (short head)	Serratus anterior

DIFFICULTY   **INTERMEDIATE to ADVANCED**

BODYWEIGHT DIPS

- *Core exercise* • *Compound/multi-joint* • *Push*
- *Open chain* • *Bodyweight* • *Intermediate to advanced*

Although this is one of the most common and versatile exercises, postural compensation and cheating are common. For the best results, start with only as many repetitions as you can do using the correct technique.

DESCRIPTION

Lower your body until you feel a stretch in your chest, controlling your movement with the strength of your chest and arms. Push up your body in the same posture. Repeat.

TRAINING TIPS

- Avoid momentum; use a slow, controlled movement.
- Avoid hunching and rounding your shoulders. Keep your chest open and your shoulder blades depressed.
- Concentrate on squeezing from the chest and triceps.
- Breathe out on the upwards motion.

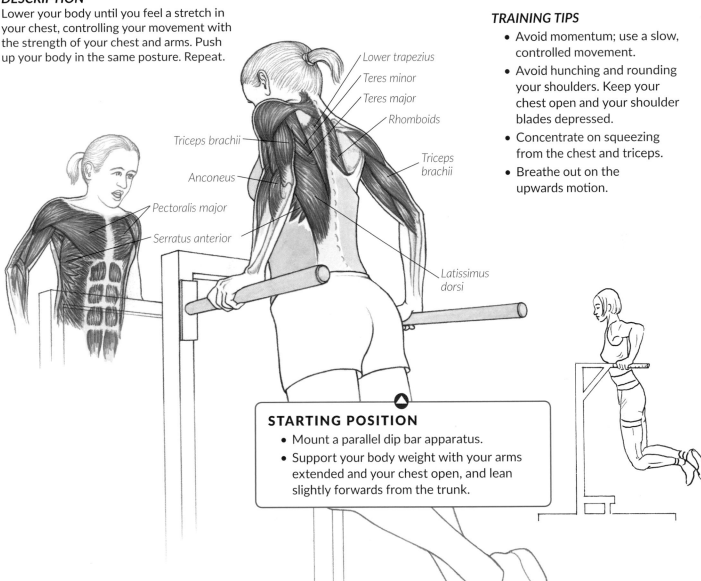

Lower trapezius
Teres minor
Teres major
Rhomboids
Triceps brachii
Latissimus dorsi
Triceps brachii
Anconeus
Pectoralis major
Serratus anterior

STARTING POSITION

- Mount a parallel dip bar apparatus.
- Support your body weight with your arms extended and your chest open, and lean slightly forwards from the trunk.

STABILIZING MUSCLES
• Shoulder blades: Serratus anterior, Pectoralis minor, Rhomboids, Lower trapezius
• Shoulder joints: Rotator cuff muscles
• Mild trunk stabilization: abdominal and back muscles

ANALYSIS OF MOVEMENT	JOINT 1	JOINT 2	JOINT 3
Joints	Elbow	Shoulder	Scapulothoracic
Joint movement	Up – extension Down – flexion	Up – adduction, flexion Down – abduction, extension	Up – adduction (retraction), partial elevation and upwards rotation Down – abduction (protraction), partial depression and downwards rotation
Mobilizing muscles	Triceps brachii Anconeus	Pectoralis major Pectoralis minor Coracobrachialis Latissimus dorsi	Teres major Serratus anterior Lower trapezius Rhomboids

Back and Shoulders

Muscles of the back and shoulders

NAME	JOINTS CROSSED	ORIGIN	INSERTION	ACTION
Erector spinae	Length of the spinal column	Posterior illiac crest and sacrum	Angles of ribs, transverse processes of all ribs	Spinal extension
Latissimus dorsi	Shoulder	Posterior crest of the ilium, sacrum, spineous processes of the lumbar spine and lower 6 thoracic vertebrae	Medial side of the humerus	Shoulder: adduction, extension, medial rotation, horizontal abduction
Trapezius, consisting of: • Upper fibers • Mid fibers • Lower fibers	Cross from vertebral column onto the scapula	Occipital bones, spineous processes of cervical and thoracic vertebrae	Acromion process and spine of the scapula	Together, the main action is scapular retraction. Separately: upper fibers: scapula elevation; mid fibers: scapular adduction; lower fibers: scapula depression, upward rotation
Rhomboids	Cross from vertebral column onto the scapula	Spineous process of the last cervical and the first 5 thoracic vertebrae	Medial border of the scapula, below the scapula spine	Scapular: retraction downward rotation
Teres major	Shoulder	Posterior, inferior lateral border of the scapula	Medial humerus	Shoulder: extension, medial rotation, adduction
Deltoids, consisting of: • Posterior fibers • Mid fibers • Anterior fibers	Shoulder	Posterior fibers: inferior edge of the spine of the scapula; mid fibers: lateral aspect of the acromion; anterior fibers: anterior lateral third of the clavicle	Lateral side of the humerus	Shoulder abduction Also: Posterior fibers: shoulder extension, horizontal abduction and lateral rotation; mid fibers: shoulder abduction; anterior fibers: shoulder flexion, horizontal flexion. and medial rotation
Serratus anterior	Shoulder	Upper 9 ribs at the side of the chest	Anterior aspect of the entire medial border of the scapula	Scapula: protraction, upward rotation
Quadratus lumborum	From the spine to the pelvis	Posterior inner surface of the iliac crest	Transverse processes of the upper 4 lumbar vertebrae and the lower border of the 12th rib	Trunk lateral flexion, elevation of the pelvis (while standing)

Muscles of the rotator cuff

NAME	JOINTS CROSSED	ORIGIN	INSERTION	ACTION
Supraspinatus	Shoulder	Supraspinious fossa	Around the greater tubercle of the humerus	Shoulder abduction (first 15°)
Infraspinatus	Shoulder	Scapular posterior surface on the medial aspect of the infraspinatus fossa, just below the scapula spine	Around the greater tubercle of the humerus	Shoulder: lateral rotation, horizontal abduction, extension
Teres minor	Shoulder	Posterior, upper and middle aspect of the lateral border of the scapula	Around the greater tubercle of the humerus	Shoulder: lateral rotation, horizontal abduction, extension
Subscapularis	Shoulder	Along the anterior surface of the subscapular fossa	Lesser tubercle of the humerus	Shoulder: medial rotation, adduction, extension

BACK AND SHOULDER MUSCLES

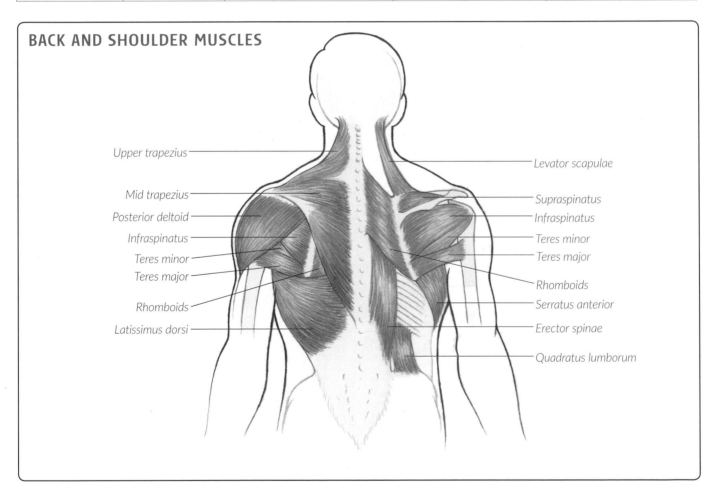

Upper trapezius — Levator scapulae

Mid trapezius — Supraspinatus

Posterior deltoid — Infraspinatus

Infraspinatus — Teres minor

Teres minor — Teres major

Teres major — Rhomboids

Rhomboids — Serratus anterior

Latissimus dorsi — Erector spinae

— Quadratus lumborum

DIFFICULTY   **BEGINNER to ADVANCED**

MACHINE CABLE FRONT LAT PULLDOWN

Core exercise • Compound/multi-joint
• Pull • Open chain • Machine
• Beginner to advanced

The lat pulldown is one the most complete upper body exercises, with many possible variations. The front lat pulldown is more functional than its traditional counterpart to the back of the neck.

DESCRIPTION
Pull the bar down to the upper chest. Return and repeat.

TRAINING TIPS

- Avoid momentum. Use a slow, controlled, full range of movement.
- Avoid hunching or rounding the shoulders during the exercise. Keep the chest open and shoulder blades depressed.
- Leaning slightly backward from the sitting bones will give better clearance for the bar, and activate the abdominal stabilizers.
- Inhale on the down phase.

STARTING POSITION

- Sit on the sitting bones, with the chest open and spine aligned.
- Place your knees under the roll pad restraint.
- Get a wide grip on the bar.
- Sit with your legs underneath the machine supports.

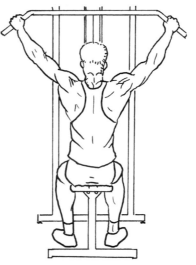 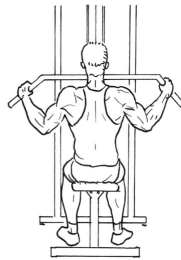

STABILIZING MUSCLES

- Trunk: Abdominal group, Erector spinae
- Shoulder joint: Rotator cuff muscles
- Shoulder blades: Serratus anterior, Rhomboids, Lower trapezius
- Forearm: Wrist flexors

ANALYSIS OF MOVEMENT	JOINT 1	JOINT 2	JOINT 3
Joints	Elbow	Shoulder	Scapula
Joint movement	Down – flexion Up – extension	Down – adduction, slight extension Up – abduction, slight flexion	Down – downward rotation, adduction (retraction), depression Up – upward rotation, abduction (protraction), elevation
Mobilizing muscles	Biceps brachii Brachialis Brachoradialis	Latissimus dorsi Teres major Pectoralis major Posterior deltoid	Rhomboids, Trapezius

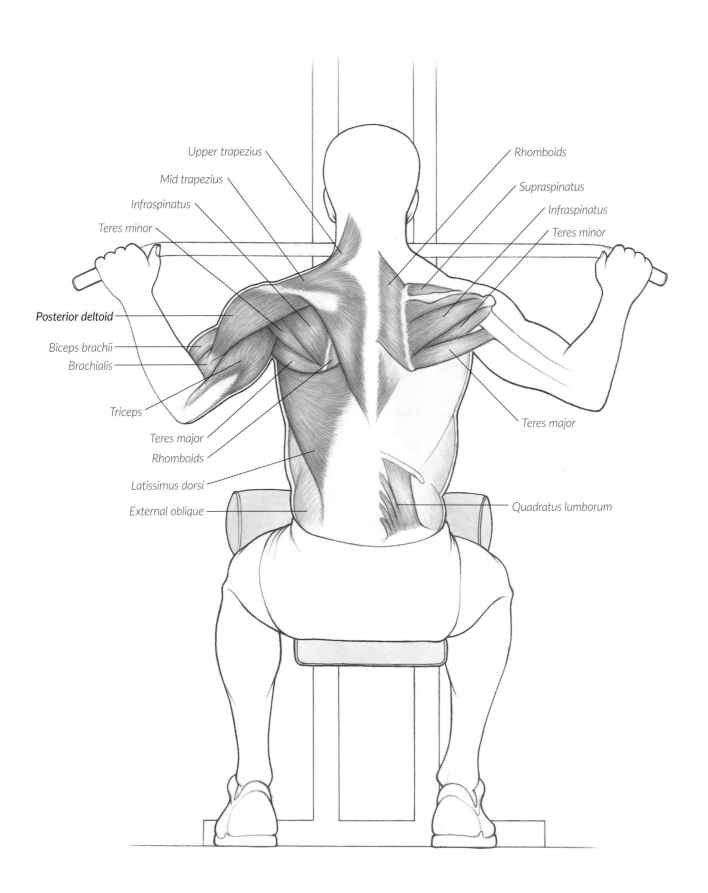

Upper trapezius

Mid trapezius

Infraspinatus

Teres minor

Posterior deltoid

Biceps brachii

Brachialis

Triceps

Teres major

Rhomboids

Latissimus dorsi

External oblique

Rhomboids

Supraspinatus

Infraspinatus

Teres minor

Teres major

Quadratus lumborum

DIFFICULTY **INTERMEDIATE to ADVANCED**

BODYWEIGHT CHIN-UPS

Core exercise • Compound/multi-joint
• Pull • Closed chain • Bodyweight
• Intermediate to advanced

In the US, the President's Council on Physical Fitness and Sport sets the following standards for chin-ups:
Men: average = 8; excellent = 13; Women: average = 1; excellent = 8.

DESCRIPTION

Pull your body up to the bar, at the line of the upper chest. Lower your body with control, and repeat.

STARTING POSITION

• Take a wide overhand grip on the bar. ▼

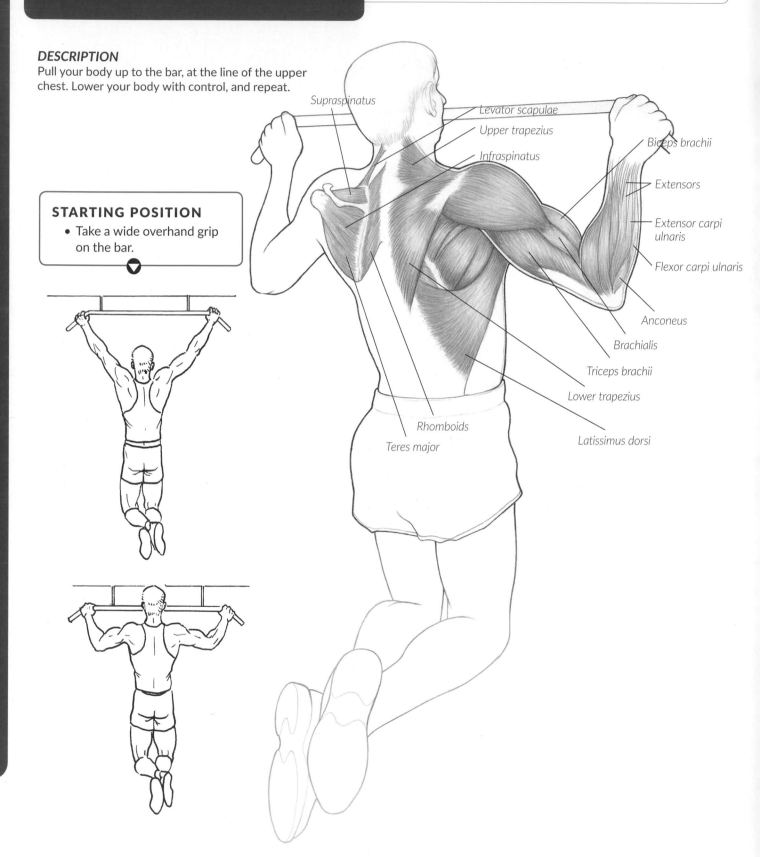

Supraspinatus
Levator scapulae
Upper trapezius
Infraspinatus
Biceps brachii
Extensors
Extensor carpi ulnaris
Flexor carpi ulnaris
Anconeus
Brachialis
Triceps brachii
Lower trapezius
Rhomboids
Teres major
Latissimus dorsi

TRAINING TIPS

- Avoid momentum; use controlled movements.
- Avoid hunching or rounding the shoulders. Keep the chest open and the shoulder blades depressed.
- At the bottom, do not hang on the shoulder joint; keep tension in the joint and the mid-back stabilizers active.
- Inhale on the up phase.

<table>
<tr><td colspan="1">STABILIZING MUSCLES</td></tr>
</table>

STABILIZING MUSCLES

- Trunk: Abdominal group, Erector spinae
- Shoulder joint: Rotator cuff muscles
- Shoulder blades: Serratus anterior, Rhomboids, Lower trapezius
- Forearm: Wrist flexors

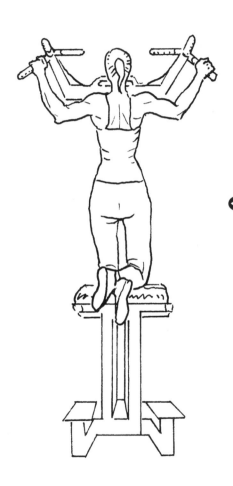

TRAINING TIP - *Progression to Chin-Ups*

It is a fact that most people starting a conditioning program cannot do a bodyweight chin-up. So it's essential to start with scaled-down options that allow you to progress to eventually being able to do bodyweight chin-ups. Here are some suggestions:

- You can do pull-ups from a box. Place a box under the chin-up bar. Step onto the box and into the bodyweight chin-up. Repeat until you can use lower and lower boxes and eventually no box at all.
- Pull-ups using straps, bands, or supported weight machines can be used. In non-gym environments, straps or ropes can be rigged to support some of your bodyweight so that you are starting your chin-ups with less weight.
- In gym environments, the supported chin-up machine makes the transition to chin-up from the lateral pulldown easier (see illustration at left).
- Try eccentric chin-ups. Here you use a box to help you get into the top position of the chin-up, and lower your body down with no support. In the beginning, these eccentric reps are easier than lifting your body weight (i.e., concentric reps). However, take it easy—eccentric chin-ups are more likely to induce muscle strain.

ANALYSIS OF MOVEMENT	JOINT 1	JOINT 2	JOINT 3
Joints	Elbow	Shoulder	Scapula
Joint movement	Up – flexion Down – extension	Up – adduction, slight extension Down – abduction, slight flexion	Up – downward rotation, adduction (retraction), depression Down – upward rotation, abduction (protraction), elevation
Mobilizing muscles	Biceps brachii, Brachialis, Brachioradialis	Latissimus dorsi, Teres major, Pectoralis major, Posterior deltoid	Rhomboids, Trapezius

DIFFICULTY   **INTERMEDIATE to ADVANCED**

STANDING CABLE PULLOVER

Auxillary exercise • Isolated • Pull • Open chain • Machine • Intermediate to advanced

This exercise, also known as a straight arm pulldown, is particularly useful to strengthen postural stabilizers such as the Abdominals, Serratus anterior, and lower Trapezius. Here, quality of work is more important than quantity.

DESCRIPTION

Pull the bar down by extending your shoulders until your arms are in line with your sides. Return with control, and repeat.

TRAINING TIPS

- Avoid momentum; use a slow, controlled, full range of movement.
- Avoid hunching or rounding the shoulders during the exercise. Keep the chest open and shoulder blades depressed.
- Keep the trunk stable, posture aligned, and spine neutral. You should feel the abdominal stabilizers engaging strongly in the mid-range of movement.
- Exhale on the up phase.

STARTING POSITION

- Stand facing the high cable pulley, one leg in front of the other for better balance, with your weight 70% on the front leg.
- Grasp the bar with a medium grip (slightly wider than shoulder-width).
- Keep your posture aligned, and your spine neutral.

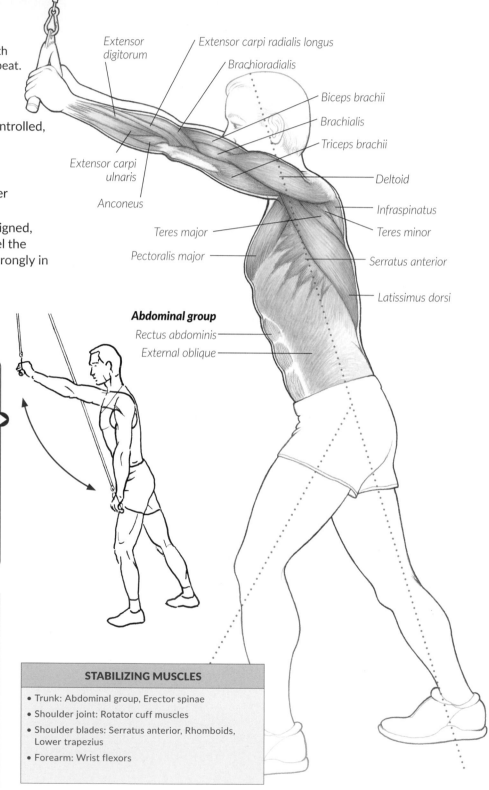

Extensor digitorum
Extensor carpi radialis longus
Brachioradialis
Biceps brachii
Brachialis
Triceps brachii
Extensor carpi ulnaris
Anconeus
Deltoid
Infraspinatus
Teres minor
Serratus anterior
Latissimus dorsi
Teres major
Pectoralis major

Abdominal group
Rectus abdominis
External oblique

ANALYSIS OF MOVEMENT	JOINT 1
Joints	Shoulder
Joint movement	Down – extension Up – flexion
Mobilizing muscles	Latissimus dorsi Teres major Pectoralis major Posterior deltoid

STABILIZING MUSCLES

- Trunk: Abdominal group, Erector spinae
- Shoulder joint: Rotator cuff muscles
- Shoulder blades: Serratus anterior, Rhomboids, Lower trapezius
- Forearm: Wrist flexors

BARBELL BENT-OVER ROWS

Core exercise • Compound/multi-joint
• Pull • Open chain • Barbell
• Intermediate to advanced

Done correctly, this is one of the most valuable and complete upper-body exercises, challenging the postural stabilizing and mobilizing muscles.

DESCRIPTION
Pull the bar to your upper waist. Return and repeat.

TRAINING TIPS
- Avoid momentum; use a slow, controlled, full-range movement.
- Avoid hunching or rounding the shoulders during the exercise. Keep the chest open and shoulder blades depressed.
- Avoid rounding the mid and lower back. Keep the pelvis neutral, and the spine aligned.
- Inhale on the up phase.

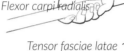

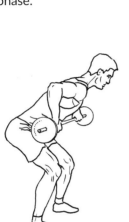

STARTING POSITION
- Take a stationary squat position over the bar, to provide a stable platform.
- Hold the bar with a wide overhand grip.

Trapezius
Posterior deltoid
Infraspinatus
Triceps brachii
Teres minor
Teres major
Anconeus
Flexor carpi ulnaris
Palmaris longus
Flexor carpi radialis
Tensor fasciae latae

Triceps brachii
Brachioradialis
Biceps brachii
Serratus anterior
Latissimus dorsi

Quadricep group
Vastus lateralis
Iliotibial band
Hamstring group
Biceps femoris
Semitendinosus
Semimembranosus

Gastrocnemius

Soleus

Gluteus group
Gluteus maximus
Gluteus medius and minimus

STABILIZING MUSCLES

- Legs: Hamstrings, Gluteal muscles, adductors, Rectus femoris
- Trunk: Abdominal group, Erector spinae
- Shoulder joint: Rotator cuff
- Shoulder blades: Serratus anterior, Rhomboids, Lower trapezius
- Forearm: Wrist flexors

ANALYSIS OF MOVEMENT	JOINT 1	JOINT 2	JOINT 3
Joints	Elbow	Shoulder	Scapula
Joint movement	Up – flexion Down – extension	Up – extension, horizontal abduction Down – flexion, horizontal adduction	Up – adduction (retraction) Down – abduction (protraction)
Mobilizing muscles	Bicep group (partial work)	Latissimus dorsi, Teres major, Posterior deltoid, Infraspinatus, Teres minor	Rhomboids, Trapezius

BENT-OVER ONE-ARM DUMBBELL ROWS

Core exercise • Compound/multi-joint
• Pull • Open chain • Dumbbell
• Intermediate to advanced

This exercise can be likened to the action of sawing wood. Postural stability and a good base position are as important as the mobilizing action.

DESCRIPTION

Pull the dumbbell up to your side until the upper arm is in line with your trunk or just beyond. Return until arm is extended. Repeat. Do alternate sets with opposite arms.

TRAINING TIPS

- Avoid momentum; use a slow, controlled, full-range movement.
- Avoid hunching or rounding the shoulders. Keep the chest open and shoulder blades depressed.
- Avoid rounding or dropping your mid and lower back. Keep the pelvis neutral and spine aligned.
- Keep your back flat, and do not rotate your torso as the arm extends.
- Inhale on the up phase.

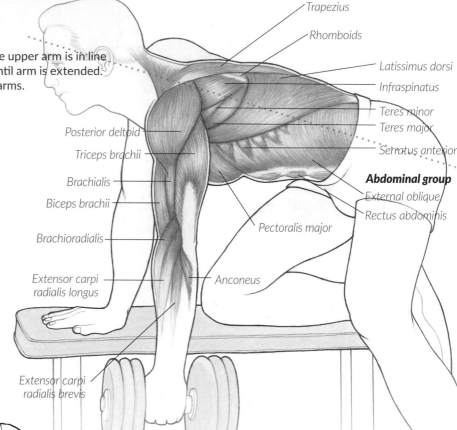

Trapezius
Rhomboids
Latissimus dorsi
Infraspinatus
Teres minor
Teres major
Serratus anterior
Abdominal group
External oblique
Rectus abdominis
Pectoralis major
Posterior deltoid
Triceps brachii
Brachialis
Biceps brachii
Brachioradialis
Extensor carpi radialis longus
Anconeus
Extensor carpi radialis brevis

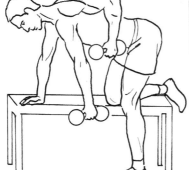

STARTING POSITION

- To be effective, this exercise needs a good, stable base.
- Kneel over the bench with one arm supporting your body, similar to when sawing wood.
- Hold the dumbbell in the opposite hand.

STABILIZING MUSCLES
• Triceps: General leg muscles and opposite arm
• Trunk: Abdominal group, Erector spinae
• Shoulder joint: Rotator cuff muscles
• Shoulder blades: Serratus anterior, Rhomboids, Lower trapezius

ANALYSIS OF MOVEMENT	JOINT 1	JOINT 2	JOINT 3
Joints	Elbow	Shoulder	Scapula
Joint movement	Up – flexion Down – extension	Up – extension Down – flexion	Up – adduction (retraction) Down – abduction (protraction)
Mobilizing muscles	Biceps brachii Brachialis Brachioradialis	Latissimus dorsi Teres major Posterior deltoid	Rhomboids, Trapezius

DUMBBELL SEATED SHOULDER PRESS

Core • Compound/multi-joint • Push •
Close chain • Dumbbell • Beginner to advanced

Compared with the machine version, this exercise incorporates more work from the back and shoulder stabilizers while also allowing the shoulder muscles to work through a slightly greater range of movement.

DESCRIPTION

Raise the dumbbells by extending your arms, keeping your forearms parallel (i.e., do not let the weights meet). Lower and repeat.

TRAINING TIPS

- Avoid momentum – use a slow, controlled, full range of movement.
- Avoid hunching or rounding your shoulders. Keep your chest open and your shoulder blades depressed.
- Inhale on the way up. On most presses you would exhale on exertion, but on heavy overhead presses, inhaling on the way up helps to "block" (i.e., increases intra-abdominal pressure), keeps the shoulders open, and prevents spinal flexion.

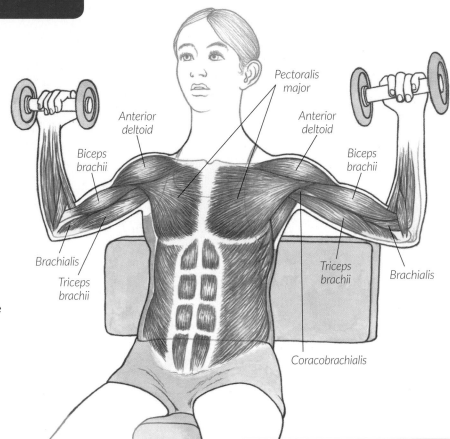

Pectoralis major

Anterior deltoid

Anterior deltoid

Biceps brachii

Biceps brachii

Brachialis

Triceps brachii

Triceps brachii

Brachialis

Coracobrachialis

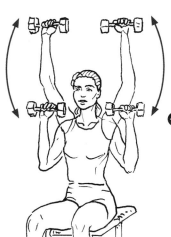

STARTING POSITION

- Sit on a bench, holding the dumbbells at shoulder height, palms facing forward.
- Sit on your sitting bones, keeping your chest open and your spine aligned.

STABILIZING MUSCLES

- Trunk: Abdominal group, Erector spinae
- Shoulder joints: Rotator cuff muscles
- Shoulder blades: Serratus anterior, Rhomboids, Upper and Lower trapezius
- Forearms: Wrist flexors

ANALYSIS OF MOVEMENT	JOINT 1	JOINT 2	JOINT 3
Joints	Elbow	Shoulder	Scapulothoracic
Joint movement	Up – extension Down – flexion	Up – abduction, flexion Down – adduction, extension	Up – upward rotation Down – downward rotation
Mobilizing muscles	Triceps brachii Anconeus	Deltoid Pectoralis major (clavicular aspect)	Serratus anterior Trapezius

SEATED LOW CABLE PULLEY ROWS

Core exercise • Compound/multi-joint
• Pull • Open chain • Machine
• Intermediate to advanced

The first low cable pulley row machines were developed in the late 1940s. This exercise is one of the mainstays of an effective compound back workout.

DESCRIPTION

Pull the bar to the waist, keeping the chest open and shoulders back. Pull so the arms remain horizontal. Return and repeat.

TRAINING TIPS

- Avoid momentum; use a slow, controlled, full range of movement.
- Avoid hunching or rounding the shoulders during the exercise. Keep the chest open and shoulder blades depressed.
- Avoid rounding the mid and lower back. Keep the pelvis neutral and the spine aligned.
- Inhale on the backward phase.

STARTING POSITION

- Sit on the platform; take a close grip on the bar by bending from knees.
- Sit back on the sitting bones, with chest open and spine aligned.
- Knees remain slightly bent.

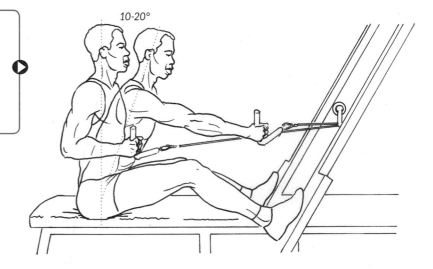

10-20°

ANALYSIS OF MOVEMENT	JOINT 1	JOINT 2	JOINT 3
Joints	Elbow	Shoulder	Scapula
Joint movement	Back – flexion Forward – extension	Back – extension Forward – flexion	Back – adduction (retraction) Forward – abduction (protraction)
Mobilizing muscles	Biceps brachii Brachialis Brachioradialis	Latissimus dorsi Teres major Posterior deltoid	Rhomboids, Trapezius

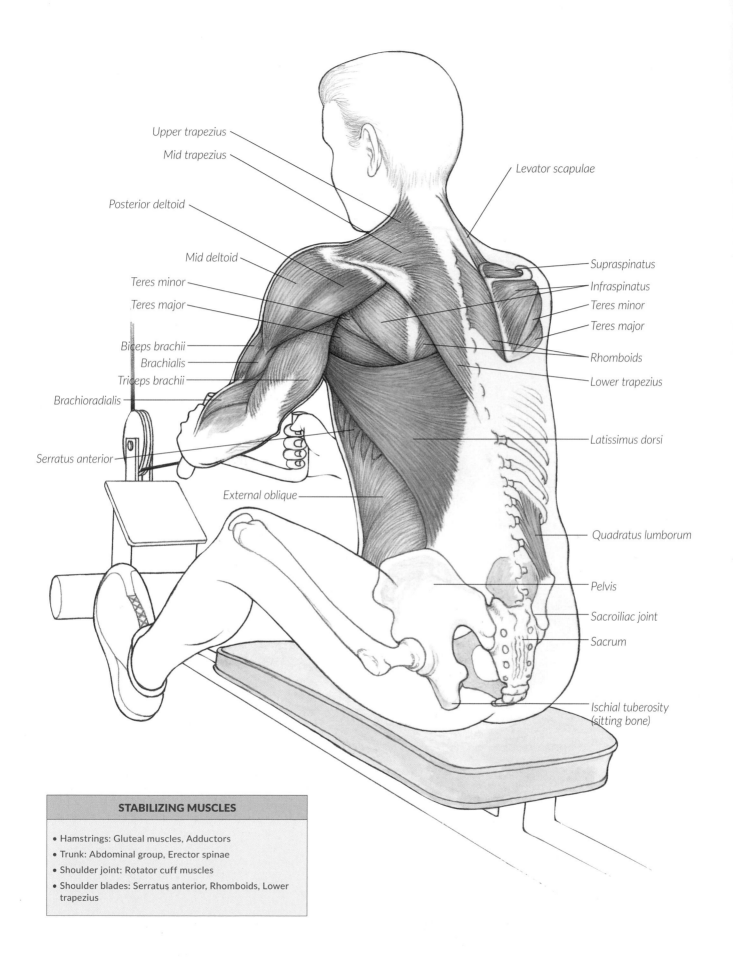

Upper trapezius

Mid trapezius

Posterior deltoid

Mid deltoid

Teres minor

Teres major

Biceps brachii

Brachialis

Triceps brachii

Brachioradialis

Serratus anterior

External oblique

Levator scapulae

Supraspinatus

Infraspinatus

Teres minor

Teres major

Rhomboids

Lower trapezius

Latissimus dorsi

Quadratus lumborum

Pelvis

Sacroiliac joint

Sacrum

Ischial tuberosity
(sitting bone)

STABILIZING MUSCLES

• Hamstrings: Gluteal muscles, Adductors

• Trunk: Abdominal group, Erector spinae

• Shoulder joint: Rotator cuff muscles

• Shoulder blades: Serratus anterior, Rhomboids, Lower trapezius

DIFFICULTY | INTERMEDIATE to ADVANCED

ALTERNATE ARM AND LEG RAISES ON BALL

Core exercise • Compound/multi-joint
Push • Close chain • Bodyweight
Intermediate to advanced

As far back as 1983, research showed that 75% of elite athletes complained of back pain at some point in their careers. Among the general public, chronic lower back pain is a leading cause of disability. This exercise can be used in a rehabilitation program for lower back injury, and is an excellent preventative exercise for this condition.

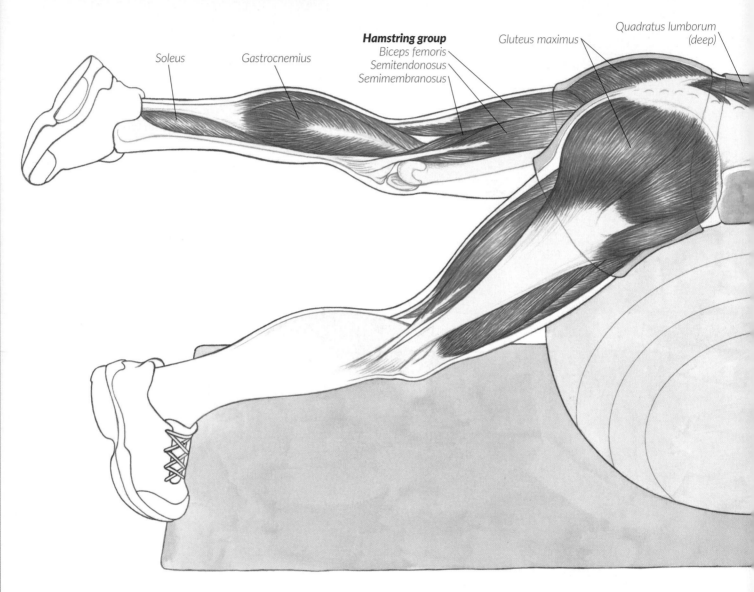

Soleus   Gastrocnemius   **Hamstring group** / Biceps femoris / Semitendonosus / Semimembranosus   Gluteus maximus   Quadratus lumborum (deep)

ANALYSIS OF MOVEMENT	JOINT 1	JOINT 2
Joints	Shoulder	Hip
Joint movement	Up – flexion Down – extension	Up – extension Down – flexion
Mobilizing muscles	Posterior deltoid	Gluteus maximus Hamstring group

STABILIZING MUSCLES

- Muscles in opposing arm (mainly triceps) and leg
- Trunk: Abdominal group, Quadratus lumborum, Erector spinae, Adductor group, Gluteus medius and minimus
- Shoulder joint: Rotator cuff muscles
- Shoulder blades: Serratus anterior, Rhomboids, Lower trapezius
- Neck: Splenius capitus and cervicis

DESCRIPTION

Maintaining stabilization and alignment, slowly lift the left leg and right arm simultaneously, until they are horizontal. Pause, then slowly return. Repeat on the opposite side with the other arm and leg.

TRAINING TIPS

- Avoid momentum; use a slow, controlled, full range of movement.
- Avoid rounding, arching, or twisting the mid and lower back. Keep the pelvis neutral and the spine aligned.
- Keep the legs relaxed, and push slightly forward from the waist into the ball.
- Keep the chest open and shoulder blades depressed.
- If you cannot stabilize the trunk, do the exercise while lying prone, or work the arms and legs separately.
- Inhale on the up phase.

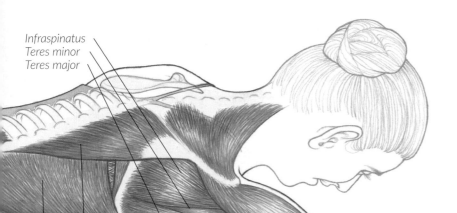

Infraspinatus
Teres minor
Teres major

Trapezius

Latissimus dorsi

Posterior deltoid

Biceps brachii

Brachialis

Brachioradialis

STARTING POSITION

- Lie prone on a stability ball (the ball should be at waist level). Place hands directly under shoulders, with knees bent and feet on the floor shoulder-width apart. A slightly smaller ball than normal is best.
- Maintain neutral spine, and engage abdominal stabilization, pulling navel toward the spine.
- Keep chest open. Aim to depress and widen the shoulder blades against the back, activating the Serratus anterior.

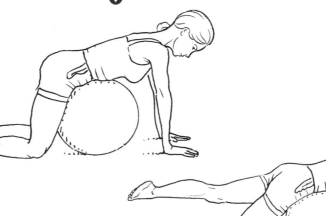

BACK EXTENSION APPARATUS

Auxillary exercise • Compound/multi-joint •
Pull • Open chain • Bodyweight
• Intermediate to advanced

The back extension apparatus allows for 2 different but equally effective exercises for the back and hip muscles. Folding the arms across the chest, as shown in one variation, makes the exercises harder. CAUTION: Do not attempt this without supervision if you suffer from lower back problems.

DESCRIPTION

VERSION 1 (this page): Lower your body to the ground by flexing at the waist, keeping your back straight. Return by raising your body until your trunk is parallel with your legs. Repeat.

VERSION 2 (facing page): Lower your body to the ground by rounding your spine and then flexing your hips. The emphasis here is on the spinal movement. Return in reverse order and repeat.

TRAINING TIPS

- Avoid momentum; use a slow, controlled, full range of movement.
- Engage abdominal stabilization, pulling your navel in toward your spine.
- Inhale on the up phase.

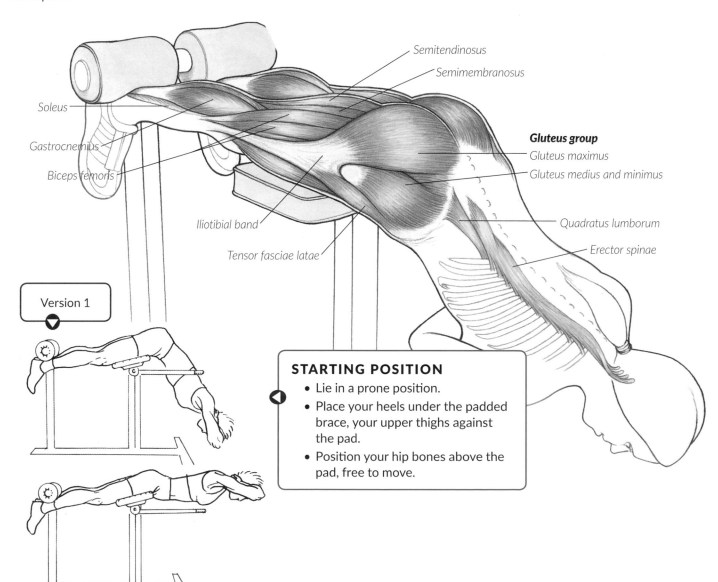

Semitendinosus

Semimembranosus

Soleus

Gastrocnemius

Biceps femoris

Gluteus group
Gluteus maximus
Gluteus medius and minimus

Quadratus lumborum

Erector spinae

Iliotibial band

Tensor fasciae latae

Version 1

STARTING POSITION

- Lie in a prone position.
- Place your heels under the padded brace, your upper thighs against the pad.
- Position your hip bones above the pad, free to move.

NEW ANATOMY FOR STRENGTH AND FITNESS TRAINING

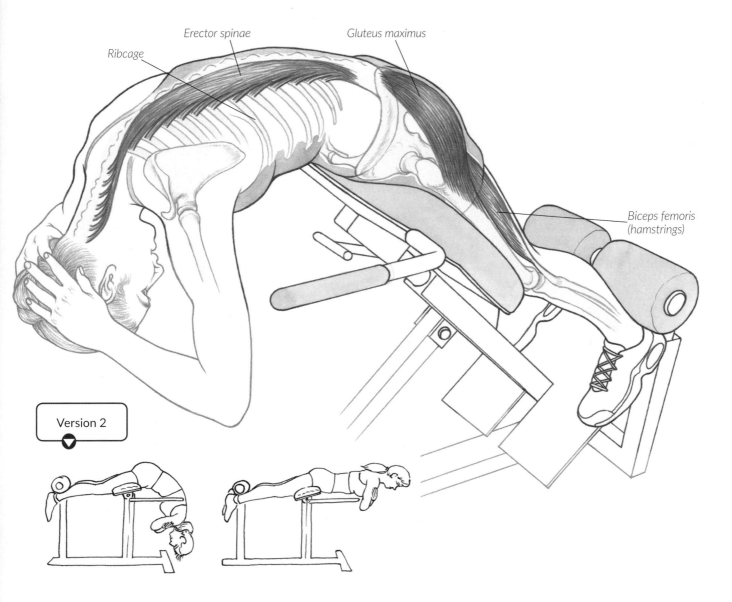

Erector spinae

Ribcage

Gluteus maximus

Biceps femoris (hamstrings)

Version 2

STABILIZING MUSCLES

Version 1
- Legs: Rectus femoris
- Trunk: Abdominal group, Erector spinae
- Shoulder blades: Serratus anterior, Rhomboids, Lower trapezius
- Neck: Splenius capitus and cervicis

Version 2
- Legs: Hamstrings, Gluteal muscles, Adductors, Rectus femoris
- Trunk: Abdominal group, Erector spinae
- Neck: Splenius capitus and cervicis

ANALYSIS OF MOVEMENT	JOINT 1	JOINT 2	JOINT 3
	VERSION 1	**VERSION 2**	
Joints	Hips	Spine	Hips
Joint movement	Up – extension Down – flexion	Up – extension Down – flexion	Up – extension Down – flexion
Mobilizing muscles	Gluteus maximus Hamstring group	Erector spinae	Gluteus maximus Hamstring group

DIFFICULTY   INTERMEDIATE to ADVANCED

PRONE BACK EXTENSION ON BALL

Auxiliary exercise • Compound/ multi-joint • Pull • Open chain • Bodyweight • Intermediate to advanced

The original manufacturing birthplace of the gym equipment known as a "stability ball" was at Consani plastics in Italy in the early 1960s.

DESCRIPTION

Without the ball moving, extend your upper body up from your hips. The emphasis is on the spinal movement. Return and repeat. To make the exercise easier, position the ball under your waist. To make it harder, place the ball under your buttocks, or put your arms behind your head.

TRAINING TIPS

- Avoid momentum; use a slow, controlled, full range of movement.
- Inhale on the up phase.

ANALYSIS OF MOVEMENT	JOINT 1
Joints	Spine
Joint movement	Up – extension Down – flexion
Mobilizing muscles	Erector spinae

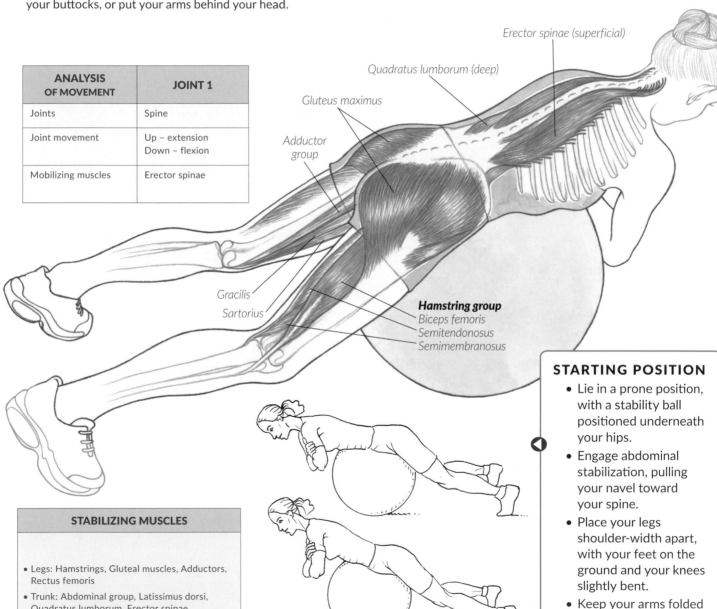

Erector spinae (superficial)

Quadratus lumborum (deep)

Gluteus maximus

Adductor group

Gracilis

Sartorius

Hamstring group
Biceps femoris
Semitendonosus
Semimembranosus

STARTING POSITION

- Lie in a prone position, with a stability ball positioned underneath your hips.
- Engage abdominal stabilization, pulling your navel toward your spine.
- Place your legs shoulder-width apart, with your feet on the ground and your knees slightly bent.
- Keep your arms folded across your chest.

STABILIZING MUSCLES

- Legs: Hamstrings, Gluteal muscles, Adductors, Rectus femoris
- Trunk: Abdominal group, Latissimus dorsi, Quadratus lumborum, Erector spinae
- Shoulder blades: Serratus anterior, Rhomboids, Lower trapezius
- Neck: Splenius capitus and cervicis

DIFFICULTY **INTERMEDIATE to ADVANCED**

SEATED BENT-OVER DUMBBELL RAISES ON BALL

Auxiliary exercise with significant stabilization emphasis • Isolated/single joint • Pull • Close chain • Dumbbell • Intermediate to advanced

The Posterior Deltoid is often overlooked in strength-training programs. This is an ideal exercise to include in a training program to fill this gap.

DESCRIPTION

Maintaining a fixed elbow angle of 10°–20°, raise your arms perpendicularly to your trunk, to shoulder height. Your elbows will be above the line of your wrists. Lower and repeat.

TRAINING TIPS

- Avoid momentum, especially lifting the trunk. Use a slow, controlled, full range of movement.
- Keep your chest and shoulders open. Aim to depress and widen your shoulder blades against your back.
- Doing the exercise with heavier weights and bent elbows is deceiving. By bending your elbows, you shorten the effective lever, compensating for additional weight being lifted.
- Inhale on the up phase.

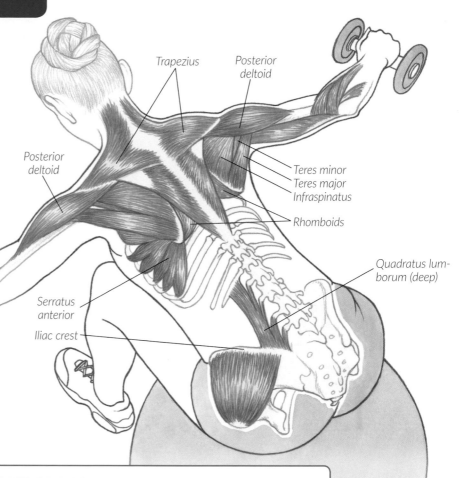

Trapezius
Posterior deltoid
Posterior deltoid
Teres minor
Teres major
Infraspinatus
Rhomboids
Quadratus lumborum (deep)
Serratus anterior
Iliac crest

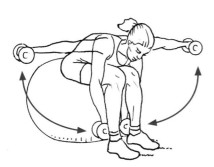

STARTING POSITION

- Sit with your sitting bones centered on a stability ball. A slightly smaller ball than normal is best.
- Position your feet further forward than your knees.
- Bring your trunk forward to rest on your knees, as close to horizontal as possible.
- Hold the dumbbells at your sides, under your legs.

ANALYSIS OF MOVEMENT	JOINT 1	JOINT 2
Joints	Shoulder	Scapula
Joint movement	Up – horizontal abduction Down – horizontal adduction	Up – adduction (retraction) Down – abduction (protraction)
Mobilizing muscles	Posterior deltoid	Rhomboids Trapezius

STABILIZING MUSCLES

- Trunk: Abdominal group
- Hips: Gluteus medius and minimus, Adductor group, Quadratus lumborum
- Shoulder joints: Rotator cuff muscles
- Shoulder blades: Serratus anterior, Rhomboids, Trapezius
- Forearms: Wrist extensors
- Neck: Splenius capitus and cervicis

UPRIGHT ROWS WITH EZ BAR

Core • Compound/multi-joint • Pull • Open chain • Barbell • Intermediate to advanced

This traditional shoulder exercise uses the EZ bar. However, as there is a potential risk of shoulder impingement, it may be contraindicated for people with anterior shoulder problems.

DESCRIPTION

Pull the bar up to upper chest height, leading from the elbows. Lower and repeat.

TRAINING TIPS

- Avoid arching from the lower back or at the neck.
- Use a slow, controlled, full range of movement.
- Avoid hunching or rounding the shoulders. Keep the chest open and shoulder blades depressed and retracted.
- Inhale on the up phase.

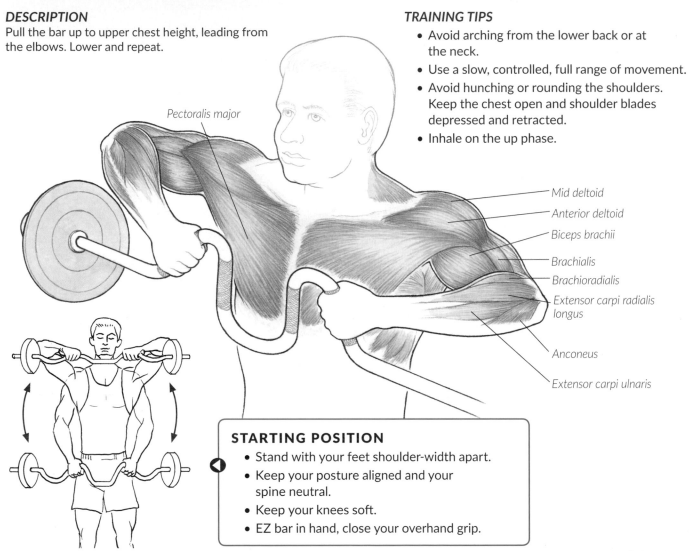

Pectoralis major

Mid deltoid

Anterior deltoid

Biceps brachii

Brachialis

Brachioradialis

Extensor carpi radialis longus

Anconeus

Extensor carpi ulnaris

STARTING POSITION

- Stand with your feet shoulder-width apart.
- Keep your posture aligned and your spine neutral.
- Keep your knees soft.
- EZ bar in hand, close your overhand grip.

ANALYSIS OF MOVEMENT	JOINT 1	JOINT 2	JOINT 3
Joints	Elbow	Shoulder	Scapula
Joint movement	Up – flexion Down – extension	Up – abduction, internal rotation Down – adduction, external rotation	Up – upward rotation Down – downward rotation
Mobilizing muscles	Biceps brachii Brachialis Brachioradialis	Deltoid (emphasis on anterior and lateral aspect)	Trapezius Rhomboids Serratus anterior

STABILIZING MUSCLES

- General leg muscles
- Trunk: Abdominal group, Erector spinae
- Shoulder joint: Rotator cuff muscles
- Shoulder blades: Serratus anterior, Rhomboids, Trapezius
- Forearm: Wrist extensors

ROTATOR CUFF STABILIZATION WITH THERABAND

Auxiliary exercise • Isolation single joint • Pull • Close chain • TheraBand® • Beginner to advanced

Rotator cuff weakness and imbalance is often a limiting factor in training performance, and predisposes many common injury syndromes. Usually, there is weakness of the lateral rotators (Supraspinatus, Infraspinatus, and Teres minor), tightness of the medial rotator (Subscapularis), and poor stabilization in general.

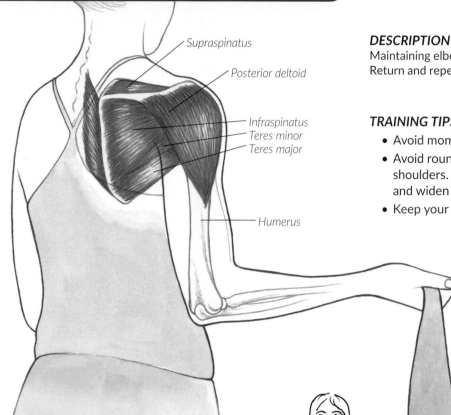

Supraspinatus

Posterior deltoid

Infraspinatus
Teres minor
Teres major

Humerus

DESCRIPTION
Maintaining elbow flexion, laterally rotate your shoulders. Return and repeat.

TRAINING TIPS
- Avoid momentum; use a slow, controlled motion.
- Avoid rounding your chest and hunching your shoulders. Keep your chest open, and aim to depress and widen your shoulder blades against your back.
- Keep your elbows at your sides.

ANALYSIS OF MOVEMENT	JOINT 1
Joints	Shoulder
Joint movement	Out – lateral rotation In – medial rotation
Mobilizing muscles	Infraspinatus Supraspinatus Teres minor Posterior deltoid

STABILIZING MUSCLES

- Trunk: Abdominal group, Erector spinae
- Shoulder blades: Serratus anterior, Rhomboids, Trapezius
- Forearms: Wrist flexors

STARTING POSITION
- Place one foot in front of the other, shoulder-width apart. Keep the knees soft.
- Keep your posture aligned, maintaining a neutral spine.
- Hold one end of the TheraBand in one hand, with your elbow flexed at 90°. Anchor the other end in your other hand, held at the same height.

WOMEN-SPECIFIC TRAINING TIP – UNSTABLE SHOULDERS
The shoulder joint is the most mobile of all ball-and-socket joints, making it susceptible to injury, especially when the arm is extended and abducted above 90°. In women, weakness of these muscles will predispose dislocation and neck pain in overhead exercises. If you are at risk, use rotator cuff exercises to build up better shoulder joint stability and leave overhead presses to the intermediate stage. Also start with moderate repetitions and sets, and progress slowly.

Arms

Major muscles of the forearm

(Note: For purposes of simplicity, some significant muscles are not detailed here. Rotator cuff muscles are listed on page 111.)

NAME	JOINTS CROSSED	ORIGIN	INSERTION	JOINT
Wrist flexor group				
Flexor carpi radialis	Wrist	Medial epicondyle of the humerus	Anterior surface (palm side) of the 2nd and 3rd metacarpals	Wrist: flexion; abduction (also assists elbow flexion)
Flexor carpi ulnaris	Wrist	Medial epicondyle of the humerus, posterior proximal ulna	Base of the 5th metacarpal, pisiform, and hamate bones	Wrist: flexion; adduction (also assists in weak flexion of the elbow)
Palmaris longus	Wrist	Medial epicondyle of the humerus	Aponeurosis of the palm in the 2nd–5th metacarpals	Wrist flexion
Wrist extensor group				
Extensor carpi ulnaris	Wrist	Lateral epicondyle of the humerus	5th metacarpal dorsal surface (back of the hand)	Wrist: extension; adduction (also assists elbow extension)
Extensor carpi radialis brevis	Wrist	Lateral epicondyle of the humerus	Dorsal surface of the 3rd metacarpal	Wrist: extension; abduction (also assists in elbow extension)
Extensor carpi radialis longus	Wrist	Lateral epicondyle of the humerus	Base of the dorsal surface of the 2nd metacarpal	Wrist: extension; abduction (also assists in weak elbow extension)

Major muscles of the upper arm

NAME	JOINTS CROSSED	ORIGIN	INSERTION	JOINT
Bicep group				
Biceps brachii	Shoulder and the elbow	The muscle has two heads: Long head: supraglenoid tubercle, above the glenoid fossa; Short head: coracoid process of the scapula and the upper lip of the glenoid fossa	Tuberosity of the radius	Elbow flexion (best when forearm is supinated); Forearm supination; Assists in shoulder flexion
Brachialis	Elbow	Distal half of the anterior humerus	Coranoid process of the ulna	Elbow flexion
Brachioradialis	Elbow	Distal section of the lateral condyloid ridge of the humerus	Lateral surface of the distal radius, at the styloid process	Elbow flexion; Pronation from supinated position to neutral; Supination from pronated position to neutral

NAME	JOINTS CROSSED	ORIGIN	INSERTION	JOINT
Triceps brachii consisting of three divisions with a single insertion: Long head, Lateral head, Medial head	All cross the elbow; the long head also crosses the shoulder	Long head: lateral side of inferior lip of the glenoid fossa of the scapula; Lateral head: proximal half of posterior humerus; Medial head: distal two-thirds of posterior humerus	Olecranon process of the ulna	Elbow extension The long head also performs shoulder extension.
Anconeus	Elbow	Posterior lateral condyle of the humerus	Posterior surface of the olecranon process of the ulna	Elbow extension

ARM MUSCLES

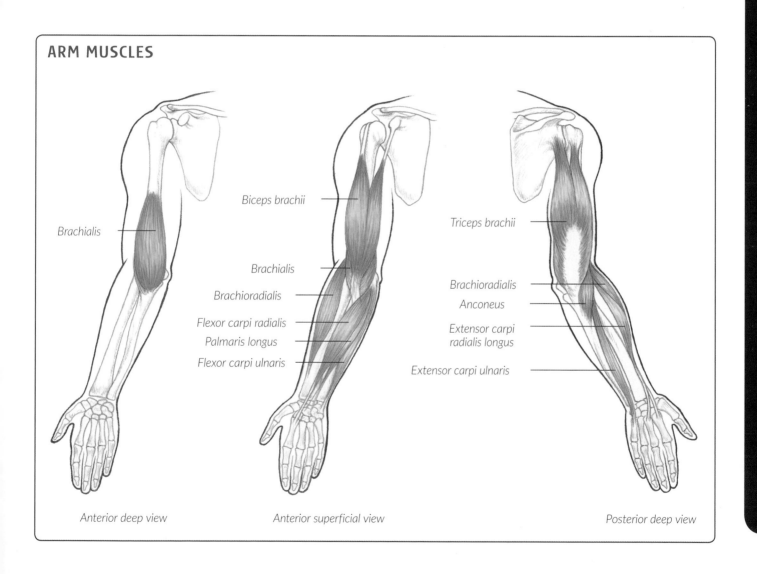

Brachialis

Biceps brachii

Brachialis

Brachioradialis

Flexor carpi radialis

Palmaris longus

Flexor carpi ulnaris

Triceps brachii

Brachioradialis

Anconeus

Extensor carpi radialis longus

Extensor carpi ulnaris

Anterior deep view

Anterior superficial view

Posterior deep view

DUMBBELL SEATED OVERHEAD TRICEP EXTENSION ON A BALL

Core • Isolation/ single joint • Push
• Open chain • Dumbbell
• Intermediate to advanced

This conventional gym exercise is transformed into a more complete and functionally oriented exercise by the use of the stability ball, increasing the role of the stabilizing muscles such as the Abdominals and Erector spinae.

DESCRIPTION

Keeping your elbows close to your head, lower the dumbbell toward the back by flexing the elbow. Return and repeat.

TRAINING TIPS

- Use slow, controlled, motion, and avoid momentum.
- This exercise requires significant abdominal stabilization to maintain a neutral spine. Keep the abs engaged, and pull the navel toward the spine.
- Avoid dropping or flaring the elbows outward during movement. The upper arm must be stationary throughout, as though it is part of the spine.
- You can position the wrists closer together to keep the elbows from pointing outward too much.
- Keep the chest open and avoid rounding the shoulders.
- Inhale on the downward phase, and exhale up.

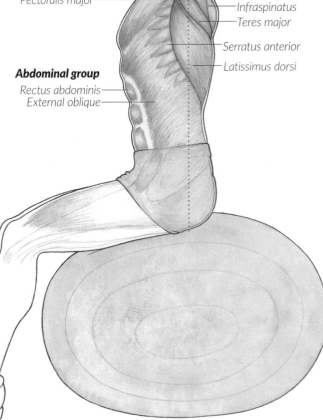

Anconeus
Brachialis
Biceps brachii
Triceps brachii
Posterior deltoid
Teres minor
Pectoralis major
Infraspinatus
Teres major
Serratus anterior
Latissimus dorsi
Abdominal group
Rectus abdominis
External oblique

STARTING POSITION

- Sit on a stability ball, with posture aligned and stabilized, and with a neutral spine.
- Hold the dumbbell overhead with arms extended at the shoulder, and grasp the ends of a dumbbell with your hands.

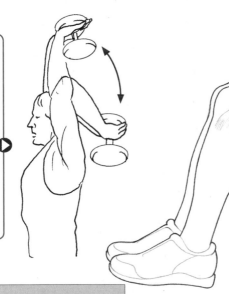

ANALYSIS OF MOVEMENT	JOINT 1
Joints	Elbow
Joint movement	Up – extension Down – flexion
Mobilizing muscles	Triceps brachii (emphasis on the long head) Anconeus

STABILIZING MUSCLES	• Abdominals, Latissimus dorsi, Teres major at trunk and shoulder • Shoulder: Deltoid, Rotator cuff group, Pectoralis major • Shoulder blades: Serratus anterior, Rhomboids, Lower trapezius • Forearm: Wrist flexors

SUPINE BARBELL FRENCH CURL

Core • Isolated/single joint • Push • Open chain • Barbell • Intermediate to advanced

This effective tricep exercise is often affectionately known as the "headbanger" or "skullcrusher," although these terms are not meant to be taken literally. It is one of the most effective arm exercises that there is.

DESCRIPTION

Lower the bar toward your forehead by flexing your elbows. Stop just before head level, and return and repeat. Once you have achieved good form and stabilization, you can increase the range of movement by extending your elbows slightly and allowing the bar to clear the curvature of your head.

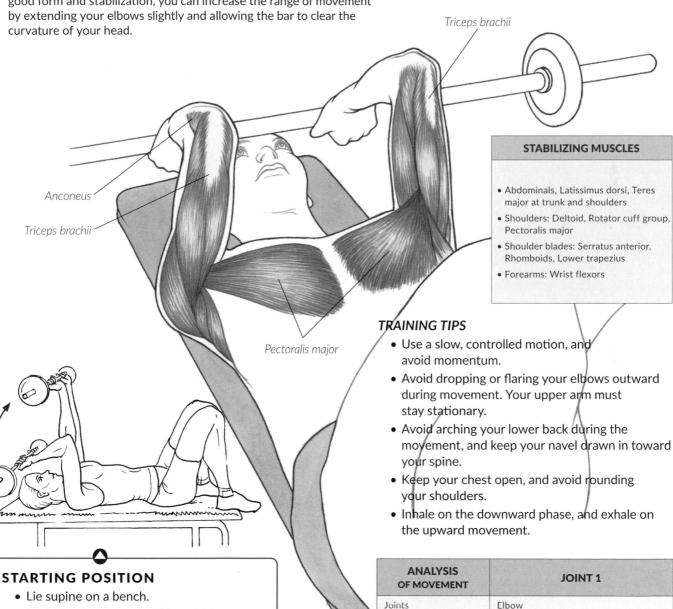

Triceps brachii

Anconeus

Triceps brachii

Pectoralis major

STABILIZING MUSCLES

- Abdominals, Latissimus dorsi, Teres major at trunk and shoulders
- Shoulders: Deltoid, Rotator cuff group, Pectoralis major
- Shoulder blades: Serratus anterior, Rhomboids, Lower trapezius
- Forearms: Wrist flexors

TRAINING TIPS

- Use a slow, controlled motion, and avoid momentum.
- Avoid dropping or flaring your elbows outward during movement. Your upper arm must stay stationary.
- Avoid arching your lower back during the movement, and keep your navel drawn in toward your spine.
- Keep your chest open, and avoid rounding your shoulders.
- Inhale on the downward phase, and exhale on the upward movement.

STARTING POSITION

- Lie supine on a bench.
- Position your arms shoulder-width apart or slightly narrower, with an over-grip on the barbell.
- Place the barbell in line with your forehead, with your arms extended.

ANALYSIS OF MOVEMENT	JOINT 1
Joints	Elbow
Joint movement	Up – extension Down – flexion
Mobilizing muscles	Triceps brachii (emphasis on long head) Anconeus

BARBELL TRICEPS PRESS

Core exercise • Compound/ multi-joint
• Push • Open chain • Barbell
• Intermediate to advanced

Essentially, the barbell triceps press is a closed-grip bench press that shifts the emphasis to the Triceps. This is because there is a greater degree of elbow flexion and less shoulder movement than in the bench press (see page 106).

DESCRIPTION

Bending the elbows, lower the bar to the upper chest, keeping the elbows close to body. Return by pressing until arms are extended. Repeat.

TRAINING TIPS

- Avoid momentum. Use slow, controlled movements.
- Breathe out when raising the bar.
- Keep your chest open, and avoid rounding the shoulders.
- Avoid dropping or flaring the elbows outward during movement.

STARTING POSITION

- Lie supine on the bench.
- Take the bar from the rack with a shoulder-width grip (or slightly narrower).
- Use an over-grip on the barbell.
- Keep the barbell in line with the upper chest, and with arms extended.

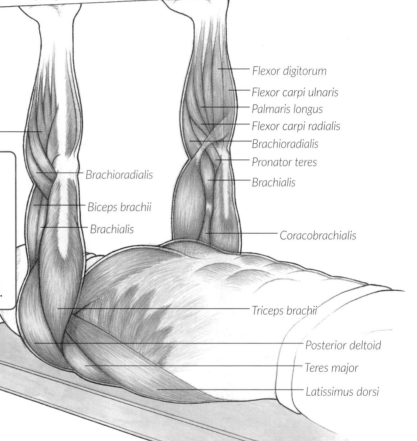

Extensor digitorum
Brachioradialis
Biceps brachii
Brachialis

Flexor digitorum
Flexor carpi ulnaris
Palmaris longus
Flexor carpi radialis
Brachioradialis
Pronator teres
Brachialis
Coracobrachialis
Triceps brachii
Posterior deltoid
Teres major
Latissimus dorsi

STABILIZING MUSCLES

- Shoulder: Rotator cuff group
- Shoulder blades: Serratus anterior, Lower trapezius
- Forearm: Wrist flexors

ANALYSIS OF MOVEMENT	JOINT 1	JOINT 2
Joints	Elbow	Shoulder
Joint movement	Up – extension Down – flexion	Up – flexion Down – extension
Mobilizing muscles	Triceps brachii Anconeus	Anterior deltoid Pectoralis major, emphasis on the clavicular portion

STANDING BARBELL CURL

Core • Isolated/single joint • Pull •
Close chain • Barbell • Beginner to advanced

This exercise is one of the most effective general bicep exercises. Here, the elbow flexion challenges the Biceps brachii best when the forearm is supinated.

DESCRIPTION

Lift the bar by flexing your elbows until your forearms almost touch your upper arms. Return, lowering the bar until your arms are fully extended, and repeat.

TRAINING TIPS

- Keep your posture aligned, and maintain a neutral spine.
- Use a slow, controlled motion. Avoid momentum (typically with a rocking motion pivoting on the lower back).
- Use a full range of movement, and do not stop your forearm parallel with the ground.
- Keep your chest open, and avoid rounding or hunching your shoulders.
- Your upper arm should stay stationary throughout the movement, as though it is part of the spine. When your elbows are fully flexed, they should only travel forward slightly so that the forearms are no more than vertical.
- Squeeze from the biceps rather than pulling from the hands or rocking the lower back.
- Keep your weight directly over your heel to mid-foot. Avoid lifting your heels.
- Inhale on the upward phase, and exhale on the downward motion.

ANALYSIS OF MOVEMENT	JOINT 1
Joints	Elbow
Joint movement	Up – flexion Down – extension
Mobilizing muscles	Biceps brachii Brachialis Brachiorad

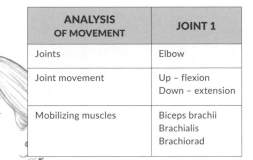

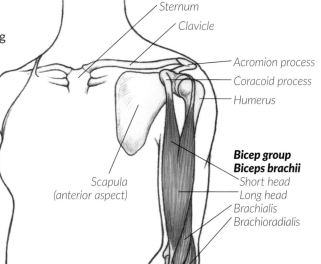

Sternum
Clavicle
Acromion process
Coracoid process
Humerus
**Bicep group
Biceps brachii**
Short head
Long head
Brachialis
Brachioradialis
Scapula (anterior aspect)
Radius
Ulna

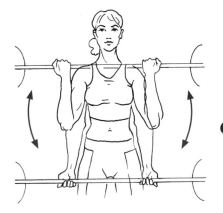

STARTING POSITION

- Stand and hold the barbell with a shoulder-width grip.
- Keep your elbows to your sides, your shoulders relaxed, and your spine neutral.
- Keep your knees soft.

STABILIZING MUSCLES

- Trunk: Abdominals, Erector spinae, Quadratus lumborum
- Shoulders: Deltoid, Rotator cuff group, Pectoralis major
- Shoulder blades: Serratus anterior, Rhomboids, Mid and Lower trapezius
- Forearms: Wrist flexors

Aerobic and Metabolic Training

AEROBIC AND METABOLIC PHYSIOLOGY

Traditionally, aerobic (meaning "with oxygen") exercise has been referred to as exercise that is long in duration, works a combination of muscles and systems, and is performed continuously at an elevated heart rate. This includes, for example, walking, running, cycling, swimming, and skiing. It may be best to think of it as moderate-intensity, longer-duration exercise. On the other side of the continuum, anaerobic (meaning "without oxygen") training refers to exercise that is high-intensity, shorter duration, and centered around strength, speed, and power activities.

The energy for muscle contraction in the body is generated by the production and breakdown of a chemical compound called adenosine triphosphate (ATP) in a metabolic process that takes place within the muscle cell. ATP can be produced through one of three metabolic pathways within the working muscles. The first two, the phosphagen and glycolytic pathways, produce ATP quickly but in lower amounts, without the requirement of oxygen. These are what we refer to as the anaerobic pathways, as they facilitate high-intensity anaerobic activities. The aerobic pathway, the oxidative system, produces ATP at a slower rate, but delivers more ATP by total volume. This pathway is oxygen-dependent and uses fat as a fuel source, which is not true of the anaerobic pathways. It facilitates longer duration, more moderate-intensity aerobic exercise.

To be clear, what determines which systems produce the ATP has a lot to do with intensity. If you walk 50 meters, the oxidative system will predominate becasue there is no need for rapid production of ATP. If you sprint the same 50 meters, your anaerobic systems will predominate, given the rapid need for ATP. The anaerobic systems, though, "run out" of capacity; hence, you lose power and speed after sprinting about 100 meters, and your ATP production shifts over to the oxidative pathway for moderate-intensity, longer-duration exercise.

RECENT CONSIDERATIONS AND TRENDS

In the late 1980s and 1990s, the distinction between aerobic and anaerobic training in science and the media became more simplistic. The American College of Sports Medicine (ACSM) exercise guidelines for the general population, for example, offer separate guidelines for aerobic and anaerobic training. Furthermore, aerobic exercise became synonymous with "fat burning," given that it uses fat as the fuel source to produce the ATP. Additionally, long-duration aerobic exercise lost favor with those doing strength training, for reducing muscle mass while favoring aerobic development. And yet all of this is an oversimplification. The true picture is a little more complex; here is a more balanced view.

The first thing to be clear on is that we use all three metabolic pathways when we exercise. We just use them in differing proportions depending in the intensity and duration of exercise. For example, in a 100-meter sprint, we use the phosphagen system almost exclusively. In a 400-meter sprint, the phosphagen is close to depletion, the glycolytic predominates, and the oxidative begins to work. In a 2-hour steady-state run, depending on a range of variables, the fat-burning oxidative system takes over, with around 60% to 90% of energy being supplied by this aerobic pathway. This still means the balance must come from the other pathways—as we shift in intensity and duration of exercise, the body shifts its sourcing of ATP from the pathways (see the graph below).

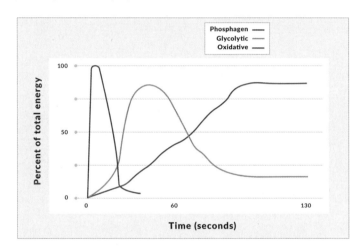

The second point worth mentioning is that muscle is metabolically active and the only place we can create ATP. So, the more muscle mass you have, the greater your resting and exercising metabolic rate (i.e., the more carbohydrate, fat, and protein you break down into ATP via the metabolic pathways, and the more energy you "burn" as measured in calories).

THE RISE OF HIGH-INTENSITY AEROBIC TRAINING

In recent years, seemingly contrary views and science began to surface indicating that it was possible to do shorter, more intense bouts of exercise, often in the form of interval training (like HIIT), and that this would give the same or better results than long, slow aerobic training. This was convenient for those who wanted shorter, more challenging workouts promising better results. Long, steady-state aerobic training can be boring and even lonely, which does not suit the millennial mindset. Because of this, long treadmill workouts are losing ground to high-intensity interval workouts such as Orangetheory, Zumba, SoulCycle, and CrossFit.

However, it's a fact that very short duration, high-intensity activity and interval training can more easily result in injury and overtraining, especially in those without a fitness base, and when overused. (Of course, long, steady-state aerobic training, especially when overdone, can also result in overuse injuries, most commonly in runners.)

AEROBIC AND METABOLIC PROGRAMMING

Given everything we've just discussed, let's put aside the old, oversimplified paradigm of aerobic training for fat burning and anaerobic training for muscle strength, speed, and growth, and instead take a more informed approach that considers intensity of training and its effect on the metabolic pathways.

Focused Aerobic Goals

If you like long-distance aerobic training and, for example, want to be a half-marathon runner or long-distance swimmer or triathlete, you should train for that. Your training will largely work off a base of long-duration, moderate-intensity, aerobic-type training. A good coach will bring in valid elements of high-intensity, shorter-duration training to maintain muscle mass, develop speed, increase mental toughness, and offset joint injury.

Functional/Balanced Goals

If you are training for a more functional, all-around conditioning, your training will be a balance of high-intensity and moderate-intensity, aerobic and anaerobic exercise, very often integrated in the same workout. For example, spinning has aerobic and strength-training elements. The same can be said for kettlebells, CrossFit, SoulCycle, Bootcamp programs, and more. Most forms of training since 2004 have really mixed it up; the line between aerobic "cardio" workouts and strength training has become blurred.

Weight-Loss Goals

If you are still focused on weight issues and getting leaner, step back for a moment and look at the bigger picture. No one became overweight because of the lack of aerobic exercise. Rather, one could argue that we become more overweight because we become sedentary and live inactive lives, our stress levels rise, we eat our emotions, and we tie our self-worth to our appearance. I'd like to suggest that weight and health change for the positive when lifestyle habits change for the positive. Weight (and life)

changes when you adopt a more active, positive lifestyle, rather than exercise and eat out of punishment and guilt.

AEROBIC TRAINING GUIDELINES

The ACSM exercise guidelines are a recommendation for the broad population focusing on minimum standards for exercise required for health promotion and prevention of disease. They are safe and effective for beginner and mid-level conditioning (i.e., green and orange codes in this book). The guidelines are unlikely to resonate with those seeking greater conditioning, higher levels of performance, and a more functional, broad-based fitness. If you are really unfit, sedentary, or at risk, I would suggest postponing your athletic ambitions for now and starting with these guidelines as your reference guide. Train consistently, build up your fitness, and then move beyond these.

The current ACSM guidelines on aerobic training state the following:

- Adults should get at least 150 minutes of moderate-intensity exercise per week, which can be made up of 30–60 minutes of moderate-intensity exercise 5 days per week or 20–60 minutes of vigorous-intensity exercise 3 days per week.

- Gradual progression of exercise time, frequency, and intensity is recommended for best adherence and least injury risk.

- If you are unfit, start training 3 days a week with no more than 2 days of rest in between. For example, do aerobic training on Monday, Wednesday, and Friday. Over time, increase up to 5 sessions per week.

- Train at a range of 60–90% of maximum heart rate (MHR) for cardiovascular fitness benefits (see below for more details on heart rate training). Lower intensities of 50–60% of MHR may be necessary for individuals with low levels of cardiovascular fitness. A more current approach is to use a heart rate zone matched to intensity (see the table below).

INTENSITY	% HEART RATE	RECOMMENDED FOR	CALORIE BURN PER MINUTE
Zone 1: Very Light	50–60% of Max HR	Health promotion, low-intensity programs, and recovery	3–7
Zone 2: Light	60–70% of Max HR	Beginners, basic endurance, fat burning, lower intensity, long duration	7–12
Zone 3: Moderate	70–80% of Max HR	Improving cardiovascular fitness and endurance over long distances	12–17
Zone 4: Hard	80–90% of Max HR	Improving strength endurance and strength programs	17–20
Zone 5: Maximum	90–100% of Max HR	High-intensity, short duration speed and power development	20+

Zones 1 and 2 tend to suit programs focused on weight loss; zones 2, 3, and 4 on general fitness conditioning; and zones 4 and 5 on athletic performance.

As your fitness improves and your training intensity increases, the frequency of sessions will be influenced by the intensity of the exercise. Harder sessions require more rest than moderate, low-intensity ones. If you've just starting training, it is a good idea to start with a constant mode of training. Some aerobic exercise types lend themselves to a more purely aerobic and constant in nature type of training, such as walking, running, and cycling. Some others comprise higher levels of skill and complexity, such as swimming, skipping, aerobics, and tennis. A third group can be categorized as being variable in intensity and involving a higher percentage of strength and flexibility, such as basketball or mountain biking. That said, nowadays many common workouts contain a mash-up of aerobic and anaerobic work.

With high-impact training, there is greater injury risk, and your program's progression must be more conservative. Therefore, a high-impact exercise like running needs more recovery time than a low-impact exercise like cycling, especially for the untrained. To keep frequency high and reduce injury risk, high-impact sessions can be alternated with low-impact sessions. If you're unfit or a beginner, including non-impact/low-impact and non-weight-bearing exercise can reduce the injury risk while allowing training loads to be maintained until the body is ready for more weight-bearing and impact exercises.

Ways to Measure Aerobic Intensity

1. Borg Scale of Perceived Exertion

Using this simple method, you match the level you feel you are working at to the values on the scale. You may commonly see two scales used: the original Borg Scale of 6–20, or a newer version of 1–10 called the RPE scale (see tables at right). On the original Borg Scale, aim for a rating of 12–16 out of 20. On the newer RPE Scale, aim for 4–6 out of 10.

2. The Talk Test

This is an even simpler and pleasantly accurate method. It works best in stable environmental conditions and steady-state aerobic workouts. It basically says that while you perform aerobic exercise, you should be warm and sweating but still able to talk without gasping for breath. If you can't talk, you are overdoing it.

3. Heart Rate Calculations

A more specific but still generic method is to set the intensity by using heart rate measurement during exercise. Evidence confirms that greater benefits occur when training takes place at a certain heart rate range or zone. We also know that training below this level will deliver diminished benefits and that training above it will prematurely fatigue and overstrain you.

Percent of Maximal Heart Rate (MHR) calculation, or Training Heart Rate (THR) method, is the most common method. First, calculate your Predicted Maximal Heart Rate (PMHR). For women, this is found by subtracting your age from 226. For men, subtract your age from 220. Then calculate your THR range,

somewhere between 60–90% of your PMHR. Use the intensity zone table on page 137 to guide your choice based on your personal fitness goals.

Note: If you are under the care of a physician or take medication that affects your resting and exercising heart rates (such as certain blood pressure and heart medications), consult with you physician or exercise professional for advice to suit your needs.

RPE SCALE (NEW)	
0	Nothing at all
0.5	Very, very easy
1	Very easy
2	Easy
3	Moderate
4	Somewhat hard
5	Hard
6	
7	Very hard
8	
9	Very, very hard
10	Maximal

BORG SCALE (ORIGINAL)	
6	
7	Very, very light
8	
9	Very light
10	
11	Fairly light
12	
13	Somewhat hard
14	
15	Hard
16	
17	Very hard
18	
19	Very, very hard
20	

SKIPPING/JUMP ROPE

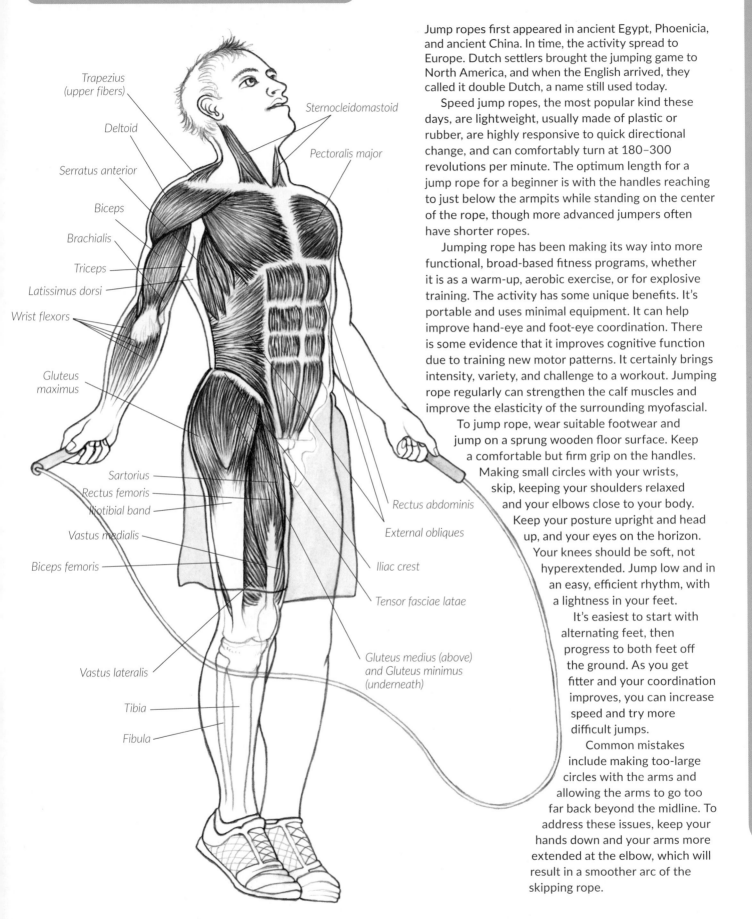

Trapezius
(upper fibers)

Deltoid

Serratus anterior

Biceps

Brachialis

Triceps

Latissimus dorsi

Wrist flexors

Gluteus
maximus

Sartorius

Rectus femoris

Iliotibial band

Vastus medialis

Biceps femoris

Vastus lateralis

Tibia

Fibula

Sternocleidomastoid

Pectoralis major

Rectus abdominis

External obliques

Iliac crest

Tensor fasciae latae

Gluteus medius (above)
and Gluteus minimus
(underneath)

Jump ropes first appeared in ancient Egypt, Phoenicia, and ancient China. In time, the activity spread to Europe. Dutch settlers brought the jumping game to North America, and when the English arrived, they called it double Dutch, a name still used today.

Speed jump ropes, the most popular kind these days, are lightweight, usually made of plastic or rubber, are highly responsive to quick directional change, and can comfortably turn at 180–300 revolutions per minute. The optimum length for a jump rope for a beginner is with the handles reaching to just below the armpits while standing on the center of the rope, though more advanced jumpers often have shorter ropes.

Jumping rope has been making its way into more functional, broad-based fitness programs, whether it is as a warm-up, aerobic exercise, or for explosive training. The activity has some unique benefits. It's portable and uses minimal equipment. It can help improve hand-eye and foot-eye coordination. There is some evidence that it improves cognitive function due to training new motor patterns. It certainly brings intensity, variety, and challenge to a workout. Jumping rope regularly can strengthen the calf muscles and improve the elasticity of the surrounding myofascial.

To jump rope, wear suitable footwear and jump on a sprung wooden floor surface. Keep a comfortable but firm grip on the handles. Making small circles with your wrists, skip, keeping your shoulders relaxed and your elbows close to your body. Keep your posture upright and head up, and your eyes on the horizon. Your knees should be soft, not hyperextended. Jump low and in an easy, efficient rhythm, with a lightness in your feet.

It's easiest to start with alternating feet, then progress to both feet off the ground. As you get fitter and your coordination improves, you can increase speed and try more difficult jumps.

Common mistakes include making too-large circles with the arms and allowing the arms to go too far back beyond the midline. To address these issues, keep your hands down and your arms more extended at the elbow, which will result in a smoother arc of the skipping rope.

AEROBIC MACHINES

Whole-body exercise • Mostly compound/multi-joint • Mostly constant type • Low to medium skill • Beginner to advanced

Aerobic machines such as stationary cycles, treadmills, rowing machines, and stair-climbers provide viable and practical options to outdoor exercise. The effects on the body when using a rowing machine – which combines both upper and lower body workouts – are analysed on these pages.

GENERAL TIPS FOR USING AEROBIC MACHINES

- Correct use and body positions are important for safe and effective use of aerobic machines. Get instruction from a professional when using a machine for the first time.
- Use aerobic machines as part of an overall routine. Once past the beginner phase, vary your workouts to minimize training plateaus, where the results are beginning to diminish due to the body adapting to the overload.
- Aerobic machines are ideal for exercise warm-ups. Choose a rowing machine or stationary cycle for this.

USING A ROWING MACHINE DESCRIPTION

Using your legs, propel your body backwards by pushing through your feet. Using the momentum generated by your legs, as your hands approach your knees transfer the pulling force to your arms and flex your elbows to bring the bar toward your chest. Return and repeat.

STARTING POSITION

- Sitting on the machine's moveable seat, adjust and fasten the foot straps.
- Reach forward to grasp the bar with an overhand grip.

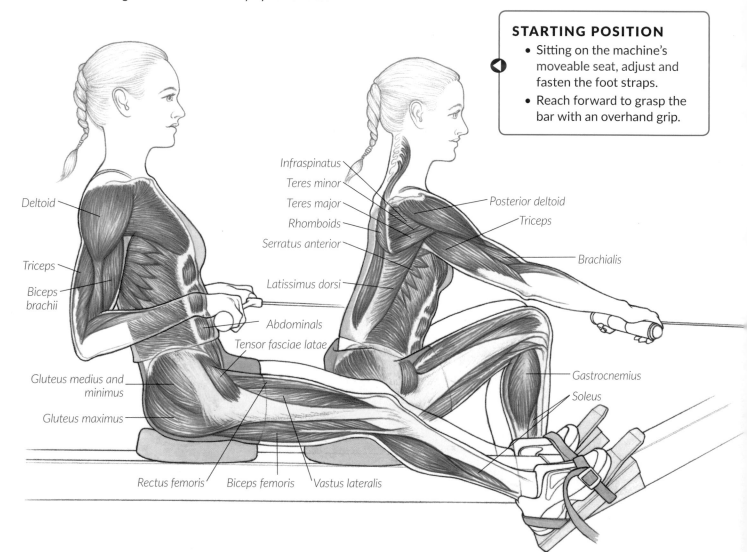

Deltoid
Triceps
Biceps brachii
Gluteus medius and minimus
Gluteus maximus
Rectus femoris
Biceps femoris
Vastus lateralis
Abdominals
Tensor fasciae latae

Infraspinatus
Teres minor
Teres major
Rhomboids
Serratus anterior
Latissimus dorsi
Posterior deltoid
Triceps
Brachialis
Gastrocnemius
Soleus

TRAINING TIPS

- Start with a slow, controlled motion and good form.
- Avoid hunching or rounding your shoulders during the exercise. Keep your chest open and your shoulder blades depressed.
- Avoid rounding your mid- and lower back. Instead, pivot your upper body from the hips. Keep your pelvis neutral and your spine aligned.
- Inhale on the backward phase.
- Let your hips move only in a range of 20° or so. On the forward motion, you should move 10° forward of vertical, while on the backward motion you need to move 10° past vertical.

STABILIZING MUSCLES

- Hips and legs: Hamstrings, Gluteal muscles, Adductors
- Trunk: Abdominal group, Quadratus lumborum, Erector spinae
- Shoulder joints: Rotator cuff muscles
- Shoulder blades: Serratus anterior, Rhomboids, Lower trapezius

ANALYSIS OF MOVEMENT	JOINT 1	JOINT 2	JOINT 3
Joints	Knees	Hips	Trunk
Joint movement	Arm pull/leg push phase – extension Return phase – flexion	Arm pull/leg push phase – extension Return phase – flexion	Arm pull/leg push phase – partial extension Return phase – partial flexion
Mobilizing muscles	Arm pull/leg push phase: Quadricep group Return phase: Hamstring group	Arm pull/leg push phase: Gluteus maximus, Hamstring group Return phase: Iliopsoas, Rectus femoris, Pectineus	Arm pull/leg push phase: Erector spinae Return phase: Abdominal group

	JOINT 4	JOINT 5	JOINT 6
Joints	Scapula	Shoulders	Elbows
Joint movement	Arm pull/leg push phase – adduction (retraction), downward rotation, and controlled depression Return phase – abduction (protraction), upward rotation, and controlled elevation	Arm pull/leg push phase – extension, horizontal abduction Return phase – flexion, horizontal adduction	Arm pull/leg push phase – flexion Return phase – extension
Mobilizing muscles	Arm pull/leg push phase (concentric phase): lower Trapezius, lower Rhomboids Return phase (eccentric phase): Lower trapezius, Upper rhomboids Also Serratus anterior	Arm pull/leg push phase (concentric phase): Latissimus dorsi, Teres major, Posterior deltoid, Teres minor, Infraspinatus Return phase (eccentric phase): Latissimus dorsi, Teres major, Posterior deltoid, Teres minor, Infraspinatus Also Pectoralis major and Anterior deltoid	Arm pull/leg push phase (concentric phase): Biceps brachii, Brachialis, Brachoradialis Return phase (eccentric phase): Biceps brachii, Brachialis, Brachoradialis Also Triceps brachii

JOGGING AND RUNNING

Whole-body exercise • Compound/ multi-joint • Open chain • Weight bearing • High impact • Constant type • Low skill • Beginner to advanced

In 1972 at the summer Olympics in Munich, American Frank Shorter won the Olympic marathon, capturing the imagination of the American public and giving birth to the popular modern phenomenon of running as a form of exercise and sport. Although running is not as popular as it was in the 1980s, it is a common and important aspect of gym cross-training programs.

EXERCISE ANALYSIS: LOWER BODY

Walking and running are virtually identical from an exercise analysis point of view. The major exception is that in running there is a point between stance and swing phases where both legs are momentarily off the ground.

INJURY RISKS IN RUNNING

Although running burns more calories per minute than walking, it carries one of the highest risks of the aerobic exercises. It requires consistent training and appropriate rest planning.

- Running is high impact and the forces through the joints are between 5 and 10 times higher in running than in walking, hence the higher risk of injury. The required stabilization effort of the muscles is also greater in running. Both of these factors can increase the risk of knee and lower back problems in running. Common running injuries also occur when the ankle remains in pronation in the toe-off of the stance phase. This is usually accompanied by increased external hip rotation, often due to underlying posture and/or genetic predisposition.

- Women in particular have a greater injury risk than men, due to their wider pelvises. This means that the "carriage angle," the angle of the femur bone to the knee joint, is more acute. The increased impact forces through the knee are displaced, giving women more risk of injury on the medial knee (inside) and the underside of the patella (knee cap).

- In running there is an increased injury risk if you are overweight, unfit and sedentary, older, or have a history of knee or lower back problems.

ANALYSIS OF MOVEMENT	JOINT 1	JOINT 2	JOINT 3
Joints	Hips	Knees	Ankles
Joint movement	Swing phase (forward movement of leg) – flexion Stance phases (backward movement of leg) – extension	Swing phase (forward movement of leg) – extension Stance phases (backward movement of leg) – flexion	Swing phase (forward movement) – dorsiflexion Stance phases (backward movement of leg) – plantarflexion
Mobilizing muscles	Swing phase: Iliopsoas, Rectus femoris of quadriceps, Pectineus, Sartorius Stance phases: Gluteus maximus, Hamstring group, Deep external hip rotators	Swing phase: Quadricep group Stance phases: Hamstring group, Popliteus, Gastrocnemius, Gracilis, Sartorius	Swing phase: Tibialis anterior, Extensor digitorum longus, Extensor hallucis longus Stance phases: Gastrocnemius, Soleus, Flexor digitorum longus, Flexor hallucis longus, Peroneus brevis, Peroneus longus, Plantaris, Tibialis posterior

STABILIZING MUSCLES

- Abdominal group, Erector spinae, and Quadratus lumborum at the trunk
- Gluteus medius and minimus, Deep lateral rotators, and Adductor group at the hips
- Ankle stabilizers and Gastrocnemius in the lower leg

SAMPLE RUNNING/WALKING PROGRAM

BEGINNER	Suitable for walkers looking for a new challenge and those who have never run before, but are medically fit to do so.									
	WEEK 1	**WEEK 2**	**WEEK 3**	**WEEK 4**	**WEEK 5**	**WEEK 6**	**WEEK 7**	**WEEK 8**	**WEEK 9**	**WEEK 10**
Frequency	3	3	3	3	3	3	3	3	3	3
Run/walk intervals	30 sec/ 90 sec	60 sec/ 90 sec	90 sec/ 90 sec	1 min/ 1 min	2 min/ 1 min	4 min/ 1 min	6 min/ 1 min	8 min/ 1 min	10 min/ 1 min	12 min/ 1 min
Total time	25	25	25	25	25	25	25	25		

TIPS FOR RUNNING/WALKING PROGRAMS

Starting with walking or a walking/running program, rather than with running straight away, reduces the risk of stress fractures and should be done if you are unfit, overweight, or have not run for a while. Do it three times a week for a minimum of 4 weeks and a maximum of 10. Use intervals of running and walking on the flat, with the running intervals getting longer and the walking intervals getting shorter. The walking should be done at a brisk pace. Proper running footwear is essential. *Jogging* implies a slower, more leisurely pace compared with running: in jogging the emphasis is on distance, but in running the emphasis is on speed.

SAMPLE RUNNING PROGRAM – 10-KILOMETER RUN

INTERMEDIATE TO ADVANCED	Suitable for anyone who wants to start running and is medically fit to do so. The program assumes you are jogging at a 6-minute/kilometer pace.									
	WEEK 1	**WEEK 2**	**WEEK 3**	**WEEK 4**	**WEEK 5**	**WEEK 6**	**WEEK 7**	**WEEK 8**	**WEEK 9**	**WEEK 10**
MONDAY	10 W/J	10 W/J	10 J	12 J	15 J	18 J	20 J	20 J	20 J	20 J
TUESDAY	Rest	Rest	Rest	Rest	Rest	Rest	Rest	Rest	Rest	Rest
WEDNESDAY	10 J	12 J	15 J	18 J	22 J	26 J	32 J	38 J	42 J	35 J
THURSDAY	Rest	Rest	Rest	Rest	Rest	Rest	Rest	Rest	Rest	Rest
FRIDAY	15 W/J	20 W/J	10 J	12 J	15 J	18 J	22 J	25 J	25 J	20 J
SATURDAY	Rest	Rest	Rest	Rest	Rest	Rest	Rest	Rest	Rest	Rest
SUNDAY	20 J	25 J	30 J	30 J	35 J	40 J	45 J	50 J	55 J	60 J

Key to abbreviations: J = Jogging, W/J = Walking/Jogging intervals, numbers represent minutes.

TIPS FOR RUNNING PROGRAMS

Running requires consistent training, especially if you started out sedentary or overweight. The initial aim should be to increase time on the feet, not speed. For racing distances of less than 7 miles (10 km), a training frequency of three times a week is the minimum. For up to half a marathon (14 miles/21.1 km), a training frequency of four times a week is the minimum and five is preferable. Long runs are done once a week, usually on weekends. Include hills or interval training once a week as appropriate to the goal. Allow one or two weeks of taper – the longer the race, the harder the training and the longer the taper. Initially, with the buildup in training, use 3-, 7-, and 10-mile (5-, 10-, and 15-km) races as part of the training for a first half-marathon. In all of these, emphasize running to the finish as comfortably as possible, not racing against the clock. Only after running the distance several times is it advisable to start racing against your personal best time. If you want to progress to a full marathon, run three to four half-marathons before building to a full one. The jump from a half- to full marathon is quite drastic.

POST-TRAINING GUIDE

Often overlooked, the cool-down phase following intense workouts is arguably as important as the warm-up phase. Though it is generally agreed that the warm-up is best dynamic (i.e., using movements that closely align with the workout about to be done [see page 30]), the cool-down is often better when using calming and static stretches more closely aligned to a restorative process.

Cooling down after a workout facilitates the physiological transition back to a "normal" state, given that many of the exercises and workouts in this book are intense. Traditionally, a cool-down was thought to prevent injuries and prevent delayed onset muscle soreness, though more recent studies don't necessarily show this to be true. That said, in my professional experience, there is a great deal of benefit in a 5- to 10-minute cool-down phase that focuses on restorative normalization of your body, calming your mind, body, and spirit, centering and gathering your energy, and restoring body awareness.

In this section is a range of static stretches that can be done in the cool-down. Choose the ones that best match the areas of the body you have worked out. Below also is a typical restorative pose from yoga, corpse pose, which I usually do at the start or end of a workout.

Corpse Pose

- Lie down on your back. Concentrate your mind on the subtle movements of your breath, the rise and fall of the abdomen. On each exhalation, have a sense of letting go of tension; allow the body to surrender to gravity. Try not to get caught in unnecessary thoughts. Just allow the body to be.

- Start on your back with your heels toward the sitting bones, then gently straighten one leg at a time. Stretch your legs away from you. Draw the pubic bone toward you for a second, lengthening the lower back, then relax.

- Place the legs a little wider than hip-width apart. Straighten your arms away from your body, palms turned up, and relax your shoulders away from your ears. Lengthen your head away from your shoulders.

- Soften the muscles of your face and let the jaw part slightly. Remain resting in this pose for 5 to 10 minutes.

- When you have finished, roll onto your right side, rest there for a few moments, and open your eyes. Gently bring yourself into a sitting position, becoming aware of your surroundings.

- If you find tension developing in your neck while in this position, place a small blanket underneath your neck to help keep it lengthened. You may also place a blanket underneath your knees to take any stress out of the lower back.

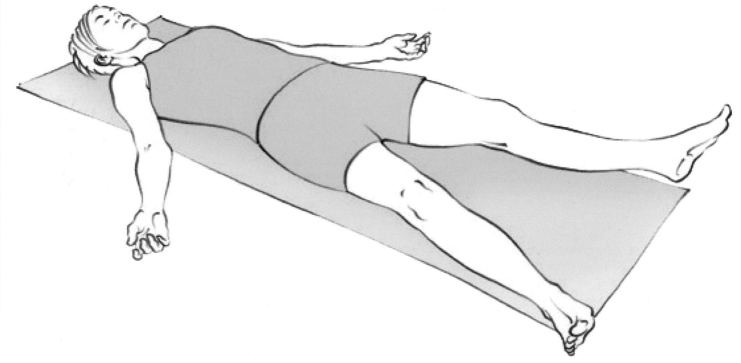

DIFFICULTY   **BEGINNER to ADVANCED**

SUPINE LEGS TO CHEST

Static • Compound/multi-joint
• Bodyweight • Beginner to advanced

This basic stretch is ideal to release the typical lower back tension that accumulates from the postural stresses created by daily living. It is also a good warm-up stretch for other supine lower-body stretches.

DESCRIPTION
Lying supine (on your back, face upwards), hug the legs to the chest. Hold at an intensity of ±4–7 on a scale of 1–10. (Note: The main illustration has been manipulated in order to show the muscles used; to do this exercise you must lie on your back, as in the small illustration below.)

TRAINING TIPS
- Avoid forcing the stretch. Relax into it.
- Avoid hunching the shoulders. Keep the chest open, shoulders relaxed, and shoulder blades depressed.
- Breathe in a relaxed manner.

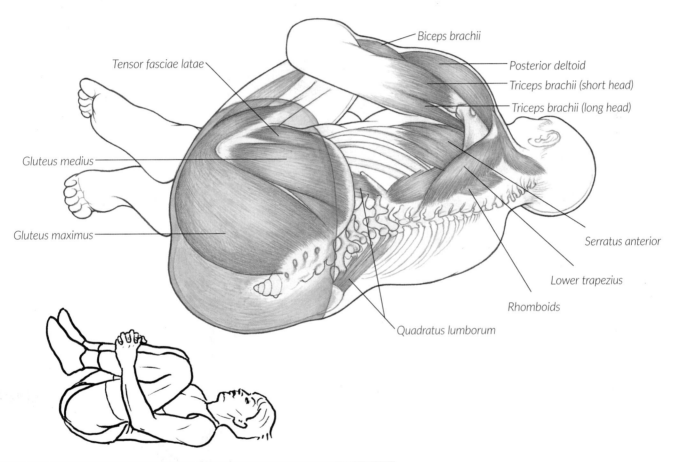

Tensor fasciae latae
Gluteus medius
Gluteus maximus
Biceps brachii
Posterior deltoid
Triceps brachii (short head)
Triceps brachii (long head)
Serratus anterior
Lower trapezius
Rhomboids
Quadratus lumborum

STRETCH ANALYSIS	JOINT 1	JOINT 2
Joints	Lumbar spine	Hips
Joint position	Flexed	Flexed
Main stretching muscles	Lower erector Quadratus lumborum	Hamstring group Gluteus maximus

STABILIZING MUSCLES
• Arm: Bicep group • Abdominal group • Shoulder joint: Posterior deltoid, Latissimus dorsi, Teres major, Rotator cuff muscles • Shoulder blades: Serratus anterior, Rhomboids, Lower trapezius

DIFFICULTY   **BEGINNER to ADVANCED**

SIDE-TO-SIDE HIP ROLLS

Static • Compound/multi-joint
• Bodyweight • Beginner to advanced

This is another easy stretch that helps to reduce the accumulation of lower-back tension. It can be done as part of your exercise routine, or even on its own at the end of a long day.

DESCRIPTION

Lie supine with your knees bent and your feet flat on the floor. Gently let your knees roll to the floor on one side, carrying your hips over. Hold the stretch. Return and repeat on the other side.

TRAINING TIPS

• Keep your feet in the same place as you roll to the side.
• Avoid forcing the stretch. Relax into it.
• Breathe in a relaxed manner.
• Avoid hunching your shoulders. Keep your chest open, shoulders relaxed and shoulder blades depressed.

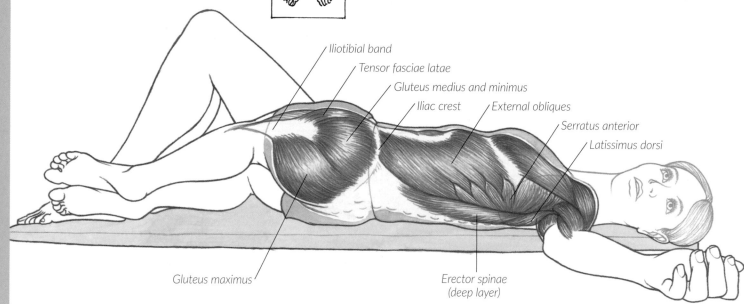

Iliotibial band
Tensor fasciae latae
Gluteus medius and minimus
Iliac crest
External obliques
Serratus anterior
Latissimus dorsi
Gluteus maximus
Erector spinae (deep layer)

STRETCH ANALYSIS	JOINT 1	JOINT 2
Active joints	Spine on side of leg rolled over	Hip on side of leg rolled over
Joint position	Rotation	Mild internal rotation and adduction
Main stretching muscles	Abdominals, especially external obliques Lower erector spinae Quadratus lumborum	Gluteus maximus, medius, and minimus Tensor fasciae latae, and Iliotibial band

STABILIZING MUSCLES
Mild stabilization from Erector spinae, abdominals, and other upper body muscles

DIFFICULTY **INTERMEDIATE to ADVANCED**

SUPINE GLUTEAL STRETCH

Static • Compound/multi-joint
• Bodyweight • Intermediate to advanced

The Gluteus maximus is prone to tightness and weakness, an unusual combination. Tightness increases the risk of lower back strain and injury during typical hip flexion with knee flexion exercises, such as squats and leg presses.

TRAINING TIPS

- Avoid forcing the stretch. Relax into it.
- Breathe in a relaxed manner.
- Avoid hunching or rounding the shoulders during the stretch. Keep the chest open, shoulders relaxed, and shoulder blades depressed.
- If it is not possible to pull the leg to the chest, then leave that step out until your flexibility improves. Rather, keep the right leg crossed over, and push the right knee away slightly with the right hand.

DESCRIPTION

Lie supine with both knees bent and your feet flat. Cross the right leg over the left, so the right foot is across the left knee. Place both hands around the left thigh and pull it toward the chest until you feel a stretch at ±4–7 out of 10. Hold, then repeat with the other leg.

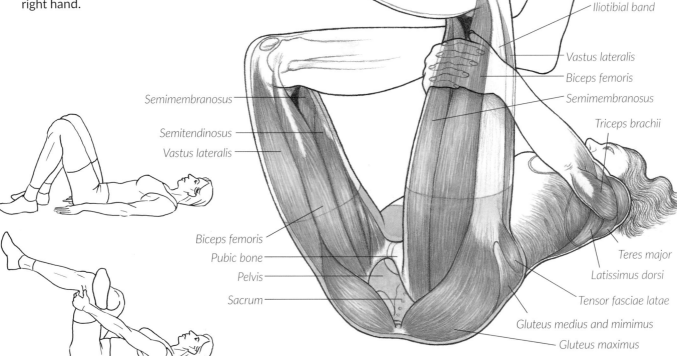

Iliotibial band
Vastus lateralis
Biceps femoris
Semimembranosus
Triceps brachii

Semimembranosus
Semitendinosus
Vastus lateralis

Biceps femoris
Pubic bone
Pelvis
Sacrum

Teres major
Latissimus dorsi
Tensor fasciae latae
Gluteus medius and mimimus
Gluteus maximus

STABILIZING MUSCLES

- Arm: Bicep group
- Shoulder joint: Posterior deltoid, Teres major, Latissimus dorsi, Rotator cuff muscles
- Shoulder blades: Serratus anterior, Rhomboids, Lower trapezius
- Abdominal group

STRETCH ANALYSIS	JOINT 1	JOINT 2
Active joints	Hip (right thigh)	Hip (left thigh)
Joint position	Flexed, adducted and externally rotated	Flexed
Main stretching muscles	Gluteus maximus Hip: Hamstring group on the lateral aspect	Gluteus maximus Hamstring group

DIFFICULTY **BEGINNER to ADVANCED**

SUPINE LYING SINGLE-LEG HAMSTRING STRETCH

Static • Compound/multi-joint • Open chain • Bodyweight • Beginner to advanced

Hamstring inflexibility – which this exercise helps – increases the risk of lower back strain, particularly in exercises where the knees are extended and the hips flexed.

DESCRIPTION

Sit on a mat and place a strap around the bottom of the middle of your right foot. Holding the strap evenly in both hands, lie back into a supine position and raise your right leg. Pull the leg vertically, keeping the knee extended without hyper-extending it. Keep your opposite leg down and flat on the ground. You should feel a slight pull at the front of the hip of that leg. Feel the stretch at 4–7 on a scale of 1–10. Hold, and then repeat with the opposite leg.

TRAINING TIPS

- Avoid forcing the stretch. Relax into it.
- Breathe in a relaxed manner.
- Avoid hunching or rounding your shoulders. Keep your chest open, shoulders relaxed, and shoulder blades depressed.
- If your hamstrings are tight, flex the knee of the stretched leg.

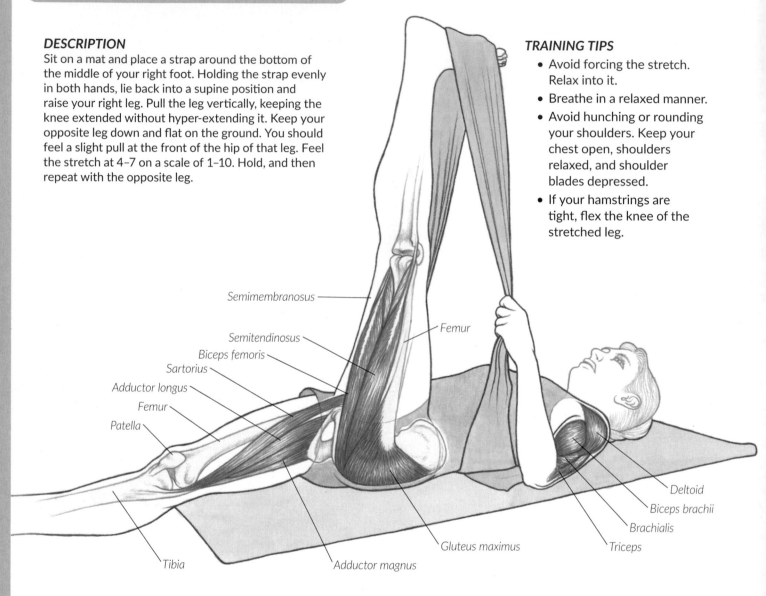

Semimembranosus

Femur

Semitendinosus

Biceps femoris

Sartorius

Adductor longus

Femur

Patella

Deltoid

Biceps brachii

Brachialis

Triceps

Gluteus maximus

Tibia

Adductor magnus

STRETCH ANALYSIS	JOINT 1	JOINT 2	JOINT 3
Active joints	Hip	Knee	Opposite hip
Joint position	Flexed	Extended	Mild extension
Main stretching muscles	Hamstring group Gluteus maximus	Hamstring group Gastrocnemius	Rectus femoris of the Quadricep group Iliopsoas

STABILIZING MUSCLES

- Arms: Bicep group
- Shoulder joints: Posterior deltoid, Latissimus dorsi, Teres major, Rotator cuff muscles
- Shoulder blades: Serratus anterior, Rhomboids, Lower trapezius
- Abdominal group
- Active hip: Iliopsoas
- Stretched leg: Quadricep, Adductor groups
- Opposite leg: Adductor group

NEW ANATOMY FOR STRENGTH AND FITNESS TRAINING

DIFFICULTY | BEGINNER to ADVANCED

SUPINE LYING DEEP EXTERNAL ROTATORS STRETCH

Static • Isolation • Bodyweight • Beginner to advanced

Tightness of the deep lateral rotators of the hips is usually experienced in the dominant leg, where it can impinge on the main leg nerve (sciatic nerve), causing numbness and a tingling sensation down the leg, or sciatica. There are many variants of this stretch – the most common form is shown here.

DESCRIPTION

Lie supine with your legs straight and your arms out to the sides. Flex your right knee and hip and, placing your left hand on the outside of your right knee, pull the right leg over to the left until you feel a stretch of 4–7 on a scale of 1–10. Your right knee should be in line or slightly below your left hip. Hold, and then repeat with the opposite leg.

TRAINING TIPS

- This stretch is advanced, so avoid forcing it. Relax into it.
- If it is not possible to pull your leg over with your arm, let the weight of the leg determine how far it can stretch.
- Make sure that the major rotation occurs at your hip before you start to rotate at the lower spine.
- Avoid hunching or rounding your shoulders. Keep your chest open, shoulders relaxed, and shoulder blades depressed.
- Breathe in a relaxed manner.

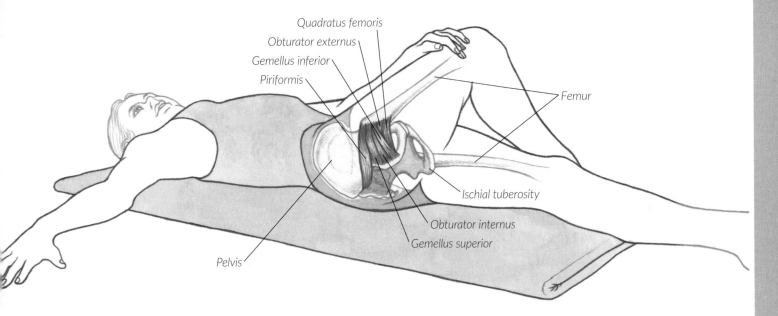

Quadratus femoris
Obturator externus
Gemellus inferior
Piriformis
Femur
Ischial tuberosity
Obturator internus
Gemellus superior
Pelvis

STRETCH ANALYSIS	JOINT 1	JOINT 2
Active joints	Hips	Pelvis and spine
Joint position	Flexed and horizontally adducted	Rotated
Main stretching muscles	Deep lateral hip rotators, namely Piriformis, Gemellus superior and inferior, Obturator externus and internus, and Quadratus femoris Tensor faciae latae and Iliotibial band Gluteus maximus, medius, and minimus	Erector spinae (lower aspect) Abdominal obliques Latissimus dorsi Quadratus lumborum

STABILIZING MUSCLES

- Arms: Tricep group
- Shoulder joints: Posterior deltoid, Latissimus dorsi, Teres major, Rotator cuff muscles
- Shoulder blades: Serratus anterior, Rhomboids, Lower trapezius
- Abdominal group

DIFFICULTY   **BEGINNER to ADVANCED**

SEATED ROTATION

Static • Compound/multi-joint
• Bodyweight • Beginner to advanced

This stretch is an easier option for those who struggle with the more-advanced supine hip stretches (see page 149).

DESCRIPTION

Sit tall on the sitting bones, with posture aligned and stabilized. Flex the left knee, keeping the foot on the ground, next to the right knee. Extend the right leg in front, square to the hips. Cross the left foot over the right knee so that the left foot is flat on the ground, lateral to the right knee. Then flex the right knee, so that the right foot tucks up toward the left buttock. Take the right arm around the left knee and hug it toward the chest. Place the left hand on the floor for support. Lengthen and rotate the spine to stretch at an intensity of about 4–7 on a scale of 1–10. Hold. Repeat on the opposite side.

TRAINING TIPS

- Avoid forcing the stretch. Relax into it.
- Breathe in a relaxed manner.
- Avoid hunching or rounding the shoulders. Keep the chest open, shoulders relaxed, and shoulder blades depressed.
- Sit tall on the sitting bones throughout.
- If your hips are too tight, modify the exercise by sitting on a small cushion or folded towel.

Rectus femoris
Rectus abdominis
Biceps femoris
Femur
Tensor fasciae latae
Gluteus medius
Gluteus maximus

Serratus anterior
External obliques

STABILIZING MUSCLES

- Abdominal group
- Trunk: Quadratus lumborum, Erector spinae
- Active shoulder joint: Posterior deltoid, Latissimus dorsi, Teres major, Rotator cuff muscles
- Shoulder blades: Serratus anterior, Rhomboids, Lower trapezius

STRETCH ANALYSIS	JOINT 1	JOINT 2	JOINT 3
Joints	Hip (of leg being hugged to chest)	Spine	Scapula (on side being hugged to leg)
Joint position	Flexed and inwardly rotated	Rotated toward flexed hip	Protracted
Main stretching muscles	Hamstring group, Gluteus maximus, Deep lateral hip rotators	Abdominal obliques, Quadratus lumborum, Erectors spinae, Latissimus dorsi	Trapezius Rhomboids

KNEELING ILIOPSOAS STRETCH

Static • Isolation • Close chain • Bodyweight • Intermediate to advanced

Tightness of the hip flexors, especially the Iliopsoas, can pull the lumbar spine into greater extension during exercises done in a standing position, and this is exacerbated if abdominal stabilization is weak. This exercise is a precise stretch that must be done slowly, with proper attention to technique.

DESCRIPTION

Kneel on the right knee, with the left foot forward and the left knee flexed at 90°. The left foot should be flat and underneath, or slightly forward of, the left knee. The hips should be square and the spine aligned and stabilized. Lean the hips gently forward and tilt the pelvis backward. Place the hands on the hips or on the left knee. Hold, and feel the stretch at an intensity of ±4–7 on a scale of 1–10. Repeat with the opposite leg.

TRAINING TIPS

- Avoid forcing the stretch. Relax into it. You should feel a small, tight pull on the front of the hip of the kneeling leg, deep, near to the fold of the leg.
- Breathe in a relaxed manner and keep the posture aligned and stabilized.
- Avoid hunching or rounding the shoulders. Keep the chest open, shoulders relaxed, and shoulder blades depressed.
- Keep the front knee from passing over the vertical line of the toes.

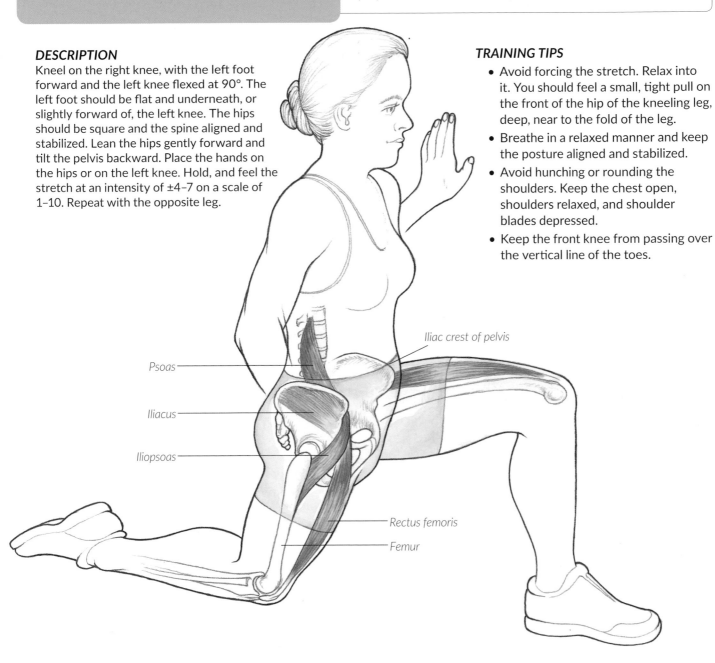

Iliac crest of pelvis

Psoas

Iliacus

Iliopsoas

Rectus femoris

Femur

STRETCH ANALYSIS	JOINT 1
Joints	Hip of kneeling leg
Joint position	Extended
Main stretching muscles	Iliopsoas Rectus femoris

STABILIZING MUSCLES	<ul><li>Abdominal group</li><li>Trunk and hips: Quadratus lumborum, Erector spinae, Adductor group, Gluteus medius and minimus</li><li>Legs: Rectus femoris, Hamstring group</li><li>Shoulder blades: Serratus anterior, Rhomboids, Lower trapezius</li></ul>

STANDING CHEST AND ANTERIOR SHOULDER STRETCH

Static • Isolation/single joint • Close chain • Bodyweight • Beginner to advanced

Decreased range of motion (ROM) of the pectorals increases the injury risk of exercises performed behind the head, especially when combined with decreased ROM in shoulder external rotation and excessively protracted scapulae. This inflexibility can also limit the effectiveness of various chest exercises and increase the risk of rotator cuff injury.

DESCRIPTION

Stand with your feet shoulder-distance apart and your knees soft, not locked. Keep your posture aligned and stabilized. Extend your arm at shoulder height, placing your palm on a doorframe or wall. Gently turn your body until you feel the stretch in your chest muscles (4–7 on a scale of 1–10). Hold the stretch. Repeat with the opposite arm.

TRAINING TIPS

- Avoid forcing the stretch. Relax into it.
- Breathe in a relaxed manner.
- Avoid hunching or rounding your shoulders. Keep your chest open, shoulders relaxed, and shoulder blades depressed.
- Avoid locking your elbows. Keep them extended with a roughly 10-degree bend.

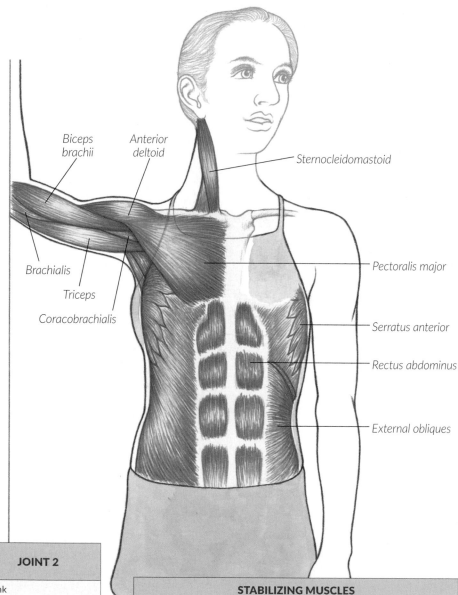

Biceps brachii
Anterior deltoid
Sternocleidomastoid
Brachialis
Triceps
Coracobrachialis
Pectoralis major
Serratus anterior
Rectus abdominus
External obliques

STRETCH ANALYSIS	JOINT 1	JOINT 2
Active joints	Shoulders	Trunk
Joint position	Horizontally abducted and laterally rotated	Rotation
Main stretching muscles	Pectoralis major Anterior deltoid Coracobrachialis	External oblique on the side of the arm being stretched

STABILIZING MUSCLES

- Abdominal group
- Trunk and hips: Quadratus lumborum, Erector spinae, Adductor group, Gluteus medius and minimus
- Legs: Rectus femoris, Hamstring group, general leg muscles
- Shoulder joint: Rotator cuff group
- Shoulder blades: Serratus anterior, Rhomboids, Lower trapezius

DIFFICULTY **BEGINNER to ADVANCED**

NECK AND SHOULDER STRETCH

Static • Isolation/single joint • Close chain •
Bodyweight • Beginner to advanced

With the tension of modern living, multitasking with phones and countless bags to carry, it is easy to feel that your shoulders are stuck to your head at the end of the day. Done gently and regularly, this stretch wonderfully relaxes that tension.

DESCRIPTION

Stand and place both arms behind your back, holding one wrist with the opposite hand and pulling toward the opposite side. Let your neck side flex to the side the arm is being pulled to. Hold the stretch without forcing (4–7 on a scale of 1–10). Repeat on the opposite side. For an easier version, try this exercise without arm involvement. For a version that adds more of a trunk stabilization challenge, do the exercise sitting on a stability ball.

TRAINING TIPS

- Avoid forcing the stretch. Focus on pulling your neck with your hand, letting it simply guide the natural pull of gravity on your neck and shoulder. Also concentrate on keeping your shoulder down. Relax into the stretch.
- Breathe in a relaxed manner.
- Avoid hunching or rounding your shoulders. Keep your chest open, shoulders relaxed, and shoulder blades depressed.

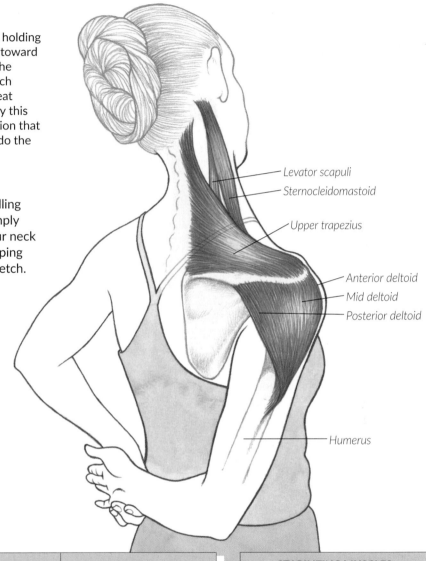

Levator scapuli
Sternocleidomastoid
Upper trapezius
Anterior deltoid
Mid deltoid
Posterior deltoid
Humerus

STRETCH ANALYSIS	JOINT 1	JOINT 2
Active joints	Neck (i.e., cervical spine)	Shoulder joint
Joint position	Lateral flexion	Extended and adducted
Main stretching muscles	Upper trapezius* Splenius Sternocleidomastoid Levator scapulae* Rectus capitis lateralis *Across cervical spine but attached to scapula (all on the side being stretched)	Deltoid, emphasis on the anterior aspect Clavicular portion of Pectoralis major Coracobrachialis Biceps brachii (long head)

STABILIZING MUSCLES

- Shoulder joints: Rotator cuff group
- Scapula: Rhomboids, Lower trapezius
- Trunk: Abdominals, Erector spinae, Quadratus lumborum
- Legs and hips: Gluteal group, Hamstring group, Rectus femoris, Adductors, other leg muscles

STANDING TRICEPS STRETCH

Static • Compound/multi-joint • Close chain
• Bodyweight • Beginner to advanced

While the Triceps brachii is generally not prone to tightness, many of the structures around it are. This stretch incorporates aspects of chest and shoulder flexibility, while also involving the postural stabilizers.

DESCRIPTION

Stand with feet shoulder-width apart and the knees soft. Keep the posture aligned and stabilized. Position your right upper arm overhead, and flex the elbow, bringing the right hand to the back of the right shoulder. Place the left hand around the right elbow and gently pull back and toward the head. Hold the stretch at ±4–7 on a scale of 1–10. Repeat with the opposite arm.

TRAINING TIPS

- Avoid forcing the stretch, just relax into it.
- Breathe in a relaxed manner.
- Don't hunch or round the shoulders during the stretch. Keep the chest open, shoulders relaxed, and shoulder blades depressed.
- Avoid collapsing the hips. Activate the abdominal and hip stabilizers and keep the hips centered over the feet.

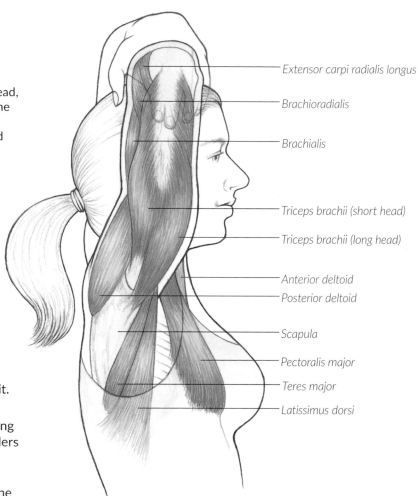

Extensor carpi radialis longus
Brachioradialis
Brachialis
Triceps brachii (short head)
Triceps brachii (long head)
Anterior deltoid
Posterior deltoid
Scapula
Pectoralis major
Teres major
Latissimus dorsi

STRETCH ANALYSIS	JOINT 1	JOINT 2
Active joints	Shoulder	Scapula
Joint position	Full flexion (i.e., vertical and externally rotated)	Upwardly rotated and slightly elevated and protracted
Main stretching muscles	Triceps brachii Latissimus dorsi Teres major Posterior deltoid Pectoralis major, emphasis on the abdominal aspect (lower)	Lower trapezius Lower rhomboids

STABILIZING MUSCLES

- Abdominal group
- Trunk and hips: Quadratus lumborum, Erector spinae, Adductor group, Gluteus medius and minimus
- Legs: Rectus femoris, Hamstring group, general leg muscles
- Shoulder joint: Rotator cuff muscles
- Shoulder blades: Serratus anterior, Rhomboids, Lower trapezius

SEATED SIDE STRETCH ON BALL

Static • Compound/multi-joint • Close chain • Bodyweight • Beginner to advanced

This beautiful stretch eases the tension along the sides of the body. The use of the ball enhances the functional nature of the exercise while allowing for deep hip stretches when shifting the hips away from the side being stretched.

DESCRIPTION

Sit centered on the stability ball with your feet flat on the ground. Sit tall from the sitting bones, with abdominal stabilization active. Place one hand on the opposite knee. Raise the opposite arm, and with a lateral curve of the spine stretch over to the opposite side, 4–7 on a scale of 1–10. Hold the stretch. Switch and repeat on the opposite side.

TRAINING TIPS

- Avoid forcing the stretch. Relax into it.
- Breathe in a relaxed manner.
- Avoid hunching or rounding your shoulders. Keep your chest open, shoulders relaxed, and shoulder blades depressed.
- Keep your weight centered through the middle of the ball.

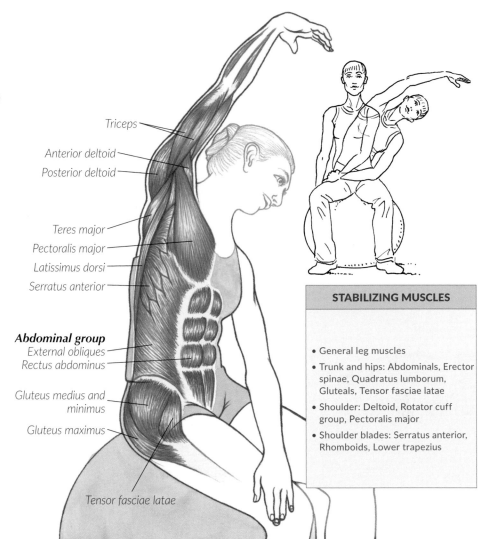

Triceps
Anterior deltoid
Posterior deltoid
Teres major
Pectoralis major
Latissimus dorsi
Serratus anterior
Abdominal group
External obliques
Rectus abdominus
Gluteus medius and minimus
Gluteus maximus
Tensor fasciae latae

STABILIZING MUSCLES

- General leg muscles
- Trunk and hips: Abdominals, Erector spinae, Quadratus lumborum, Gluteals, Tensor fasciae latae
- Shoulder: Deltoid, Rotator cuff group, Pectoralis major
- Shoulder blades: Serratus anterior, Rhomboids, Lower trapezius

STRETCH ANALYSIS	JOINT 1	JOINT 2	JOINT 3	JOINT 4
Active joints	Spine (side of raised arm)	Scapula (side of raised arm)	Shoulder (side of raised arm)	Neck (i.e., cervical spine)
Joint position	Laterally flexed	Upwardly rotated	Abducted	Laterally flexed
Main stretching muscles	Erector spinae group Quadratus lumborum Latissimus dorsi Abdominal group	Lower aspect of Rhomboids Lower trapezius Teres major Teres minor	Latissimus dorsi Rotator cuff group Pectoralis major, emphasis on the sternal and abdominal portion Deltoid with emphasis on posterior aspect Long head of Tricep Coracobrachialis	Upper trapezius* Splenius Sternocleidomastoid Levator scapulae* Rectus capitis lateralis *Across cervical spine but attached to scapula (all on side being stretched)

BALL SHOULDER STRETCH

Static • Compound/multi-joint • Close chain
• Bodyweight • Beginner to advanced

This deep, relaxing stretch helps to ease the tension in the shoulders and upper back, as well as realign the shoulder joint into its socket.

DESCRIPTION

Kneel on a mat with a stability ball in front of you. Place your hands on the sides of the ball. Lean your buttocks back to your hips, going into a kneeling position while rolling the ball forward with your hands, so that your head and trunk become horizontal, face looking down. Hold the stretch at 4–7 on a scale of 1–10.

TRAINING TIPS

- Avoid hunching or rounding your shoulders. Keep your chest open, shoulders relaxed, and shoulder blades depressed.
- Avoid arching your neck: keep your eyes toward the floor.
- Avoid forcing the stretch. Relax into it.
- Breathe in a relaxed manner.

STABILIZING MUSCLES

- Trunk: Abdominal group, Erector spinae, Quadratus lumborum
- Scapula: Lower trapezius, Rhomboids, Serratus anterior
- Shoulders: Rotator cuff
- Neck: Splenius capitus and cervicis

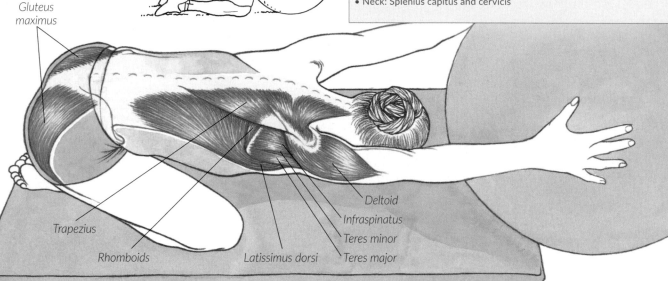

Gluteus maximus

Trapezius

Rhomboids

Latissimus dorsi

Deltoid
Infraspinatus
Teres minor
Teres major

STRETCH ANALYSIS	JOINT 1	JOINT 2	JOINT 3	JOINT 4
Active joints	Shoulder	Scapula	Hip	Knee
Joint position	Flexed and internally rotated	Depressed	Flexed	Flexed
Main stretching muscles	Pectoralis major, Latissimus dorsi, Anterior deltoid, Rotator cuff group, Biceps brachii	Pectoralis minor Teres major Teres minor Mid and Lower trapezius Lower rhomboids	Gluteus maximus Hamstring group	Quadricep group

FULL-BODY STRETCH

Static • Compound/multi-joint
• Bodyweight • Beginner to advanced

This stretch, adapted from yoga, is simpler than it looks. It is a surprising and wonderful full-body stretch that can be done almost anywhere.

DESCRIPTION

Sit slightly forward on a bench with your feet flat and knees bent, positioned above your feet. Leaning forward from your hips, twist your spine to one side, placing the back of your elbow against your inside knee. As you twist, open your chest and raise and extend your other arm. Turn your head to look at the upper hand. Hold at 4–7 on a scale of 1–10. Return and repeat on the other side.

TRAINING TIPS

- Lengthen both arms away from each other, expanding your chest.
- Avoid forcing the stretch. Relax into it.
- Breathe in a relaxed manner.
- Avoid hunching or rounding your shoulders. Keep your chest open, shoulders relaxed, and shoulder blades depressed.

STABILIZING MUSCLES

- General leg muscles
- Trunk and hips: Abdominals, Erector spinae, Quadratus lumborum, Tensor fascia latae
- Shoulders: Deltoid, Rotator cuff group, Pectoralis major
- Shoulder blades: Serratus anterior, Rhomboids, Lower trapezius
- Neck: Sternocleidomastoid, Rectus capitis lateralis

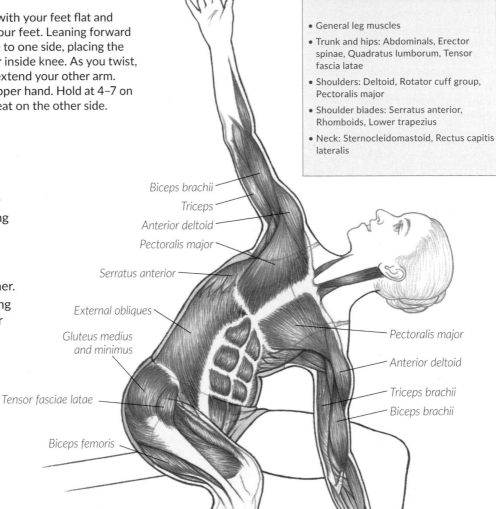

Biceps brachii
Triceps
Anterior deltoid
Pectoralis major
Serratus anterior
External obliques
Gluteus medius and minimus
Tensor fasciae latae
Biceps femoris

Pectoralis major
Anterior deltoid
Triceps brachii
Biceps brachii

STRETCH ANALYSIS	JOINT 1	JOINT 2	JOINT 3
Active joints	Hips, on open side	Spine	Shoulder (top arm)
Joint position	Flexed	Horizontal rotation to open side	Horizontally abducted and laterally rotated
Main stretching muscles	Gluteus maximus Hamstring group, emphasis on upper portion	Abdominal group, emphasis on external oblique Quadratus lumborum Latissimus dorsi Lower erector spinae	Pectoralis major Corcobrachialis Anterior deltoid Long head of Tricep

DIFFICULTY **BEGINNER to ADVANCED**

SPINE ROLL

Static • Compound/multi-joint
• Bodyweight • Beginner to advanced

This simple stretch is ideal for releasing the typical lower back tension that tends to accumulate from the postural stressors of modern-day living. It is also a good warm-up stretch for other supine lying lower-body stretches.

DESCRIPTION

Kneel on all fours over a stability ball, as shown. Maintain a neutral spine, keeping abdominal stabilization engaged and pulling your navel into your spine. Round your spine up to the ceiling, rounding as much as possible on the full length of the spine. Relax and lower your spine back to neutral. Dip your abdominals forward, lifting your head.

TRAINING TIPS

- Avoid forcing the stretch. Relax into it.
- Breathe in a relaxed manner.
- Avoid hunching your shoulders. Keep your chest open, shoulders relaxed, and shoulder blades depressed.

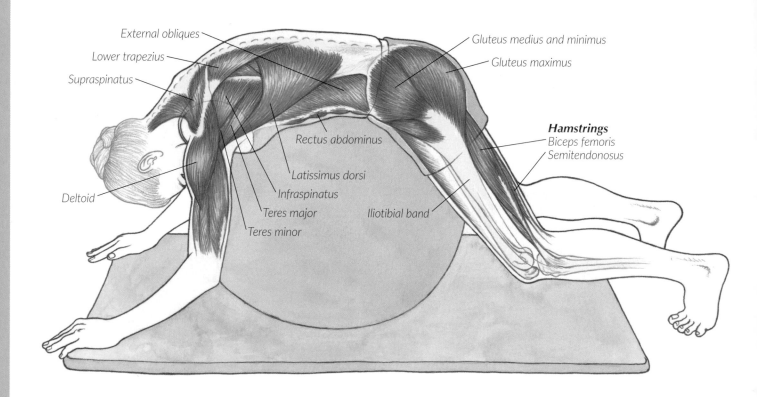

External obliques
Lower trapezius
Supraspinatus
Deltoid
Rectus abdominus
Latissimus dorsi
Infraspinatus
Teres major
Teres minor
Iliotibial band
Gluteus medius and minimus
Gluteus maximus
Hamstrings
Biceps femoris
Semitendonosus

STRETCH ANALYSIS	JOINT 1	JOINT 2
Active joints	Spine	Hips
Joint position	Flexed	Mild flexion
Main stretching muscles	Erector spinae Lower and Mid trapezius Rhomboids Quadratus lumborum Latissimus dorsi	Gluteus maximus Hamstring group (upper part)

STABILIZING MUSCLES

- Arms: Tricep, forearm muscles
- Shoulder joints: Posterior deltoid, Latissimus dorsi, Teres major, Rotator cuff muscles
- Abdominal group
- Shoulder blades: Serratus anterior, Rhomboids, Lower trapezius

ABDOMINALS

Static • Compound/multi-joint
Bodyweight • Intermediate to advanced

Done mindfully, this stretch is a meditative opener and lengthener of the front line. Go slowly, and think lengthening, not bending, of the spine.

DESCRIPTION

To increase the stretch, extend your knees allowing your head to move further toward the floor until you feel a stretch in your abdominals. Breathe in and out through your nose, allowing your abdomen to rise and fall with each breath. Every 2 to 3 breaths, increase the stretch on the exhalation. Continue for 1 to 2 minutes.

TRAINING TIPS

- Ensure the sacrum is in contact with the ball throughout the stretch.

STARTING POSITION

- Begin by lying supine (face up) over a Swiss ball, with your sacrum, spine, and head all in contact with the ball and with your knees bent.
- Place your arms overhead.

Abdominal group
Rectus abdominus
External obliques
Internal obliques (underneath)

Intercostal muscles
Pectoralis major
Sternocleidomastoid
Anterior deltoid
Coracoid process
Teres major
Latissimus dorsi
Subscapularis

Note: *If you ever feel dizzy while looking up, for instance when looking in overhead cupboards or looking up at airplanes, do not perform this stretch. If you feel faint or dizzy doing this stretch, stop immediately. You may wish to have a trained professional check your neck for vertebral artery occlusion.*

STRETCH ANALYSIS	Joints	Joint movement	Muscles stretched
JOINT 1	Cervical spine	Extension	Sternocleidomastoid, Scalenes (anterior fibers), Longus capitis, Longus coli
JOINT 2	Thoracic and lumbar spine	Extension	Rectus abdominus, External obliques, Internal obliques, Internal intercostals
JOINT 3	Shoulder	Flexion, abduction, external rotation	Pectoralis major, Anterior deltoid, Subscapularis, Latissimus dorsi, Teres major

PLANK TO DOWNWARD-FACING DOG

Static/dynamic • Compound/multi-joint • Close chain
• Bodyweight • Intermediate to advanced

The downward dog forms part of the sun salutation, a yoga sequence of 12 postures performed in a single, graceful flow, done in coordination with the breath.

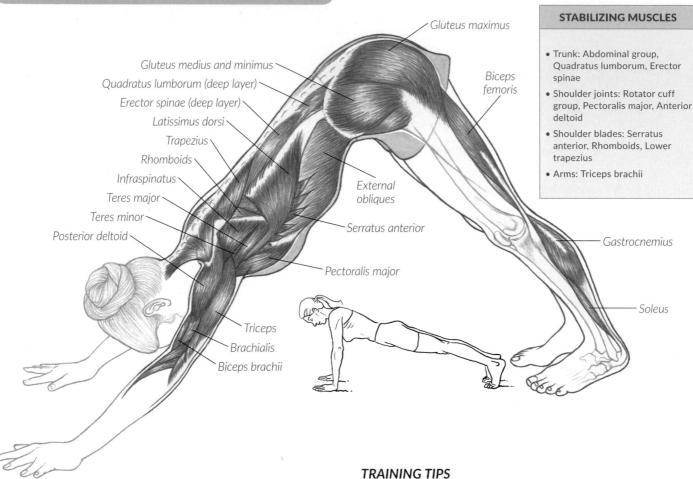

Gluteus maximus

Gluteus medius and minimus
Quadratus lumborum (deep layer)
Erector spinae (deep layer)
Latissimus dorsi
Trapezius
Rhomboids
Infraspinatus
Teres major
Teres minor
Posterior deltoid

Biceps femoris

External obliques

Serratus anterior

Pectoralis major

Gastrocnemius

Soleus

Triceps
Brachialis
Biceps brachii

STABILIZING MUSCLES

- Trunk: Abdominal group, Quadratus lumborum, Erector spinae
- Shoulder joints: Rotator cuff group, Pectoralis major, Anterior deltoid
- Shoulder blades: Serratus anterior, Rhomboids, Lower trapezius
- Arms: Triceps brachii

DESCRIPTION

Raise your body, supporting yourself on your hands and feet. Extend your arms slightly more than shoulder-width apart, at the level of your upper chest. Maintain a neutral spine, with abdominal stabilization engaged, squeezing your navel into your spine. Exhale, lift from the hips, then push them back and up. Keep your chest open.

TRAINING TIPS

- At first keep your knees slightly bent and your heels lifted off the floor.
- Try to lift your sitting bones to the ceiling; settle back toward a flat foot.
- Depress and widen your shoulder blades.
- Keep your hands flat, with the palms spread out and the index fingers parallel to each other.

STRETCH ANALYSIS	JOINT 1	JOINT 2	JOINT 3	JOINT 4
Active joints	Ankle	Knees	Hips and pelvis	Shoulders
Joint position	Dorsiflexed	Extended	Flexed	Full flexion and internal rotation
Main stretching muscles	Gastrocnemius Soleus Plantaris Tibialis posterior Flexor digitorum longus Flexor hallucis longus	Gastrocnemius Hamstring group Popliteus	Gluteus maximus Hamstring group Quadratus lumborum Latissimus dorsi Erector spinae	Triceps brachii Biceps brachii Rotator cuff group Latissimus dorsi Teres major Deltoid Pectoralis major, emphasis on abdominal (lower) aspect

CHILD STRETCH

Static/dynamic • Compound/multi-joint • Close chain
• Bodyweight • Beginner to advanced

This child pose derives from yoga. It can provide a calming end to an intense workout or series of intense exercises or stretches.

DESCRIPTION

Kneel prone on an exercise or yoga mat with your knees slightly apart. Rest your arms at your sides. Let your head lie on the mat, to the side or on your forehead, whichever is more comfortable.

TRAINING TIPS

- The key in this stretch is to relax. Let your body naturally soften and be comfortable.

BREATHING AND RELAXATION TIP

Relaxed or diaphragmatic breathing is the body's natural breathing response. Chronic stress can condition a shallow, limited breath into the body's neural responses, which brings in up to 90% less oxygen than relaxation breathing. That is why stress breathing can promote fatigue and poor concentration (poor oxygen supply to the brain), poor digestion (collapsed chest), and increased muscle tension (from mild hypoxia effect). Use relaxation or deep-breathing practices on a regular basis. Start with as little as 3 deep breaths. Breathe in through the nose and let the air passively escape through the mouth. Relaxation breathing can be done anywhere and can help promote a state of relaxation, clarity, and alertness.

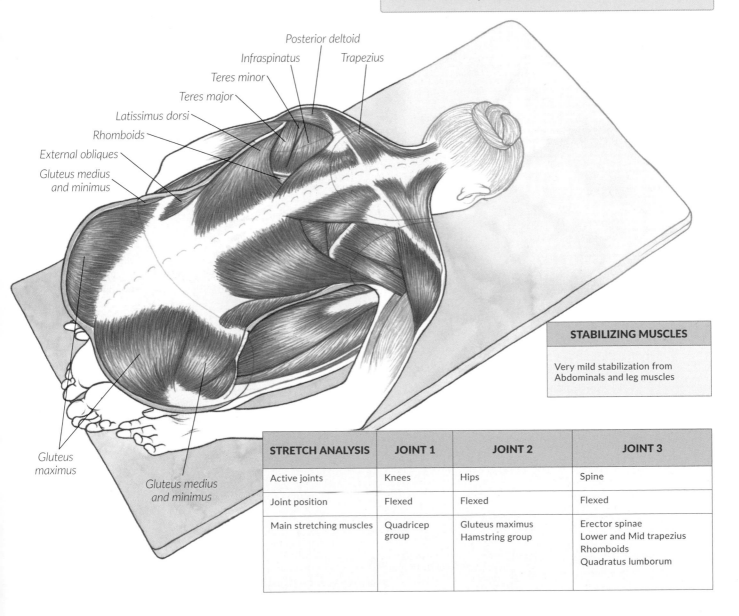

Posterior deltoid
Infraspinatus
Trapezius
Teres minor
Teres major
Latissimus dorsi
Rhomboids
External obliques
Gluteus medius and minimus
Gluteus maximus
Gluteus medius and minimus

STABILIZING MUSCLES

Very mild stabilization from Abdominals and leg muscles

STRETCH ANALYSIS	JOINT 1	JOINT 2	JOINT 3
Active joints	Knees	Hips	Spine
Joint position	Flexed	Flexed	Flexed
Main stretching muscles	Quadricep group	Gluteus maximus Hamstring group	Erector spinae Lower and Mid trapezius Rhomboids Quadratus lumborum

Resources

FURTHER READING

Baker, Robert B. **Training with Weights: The Athlete's Free-Weight Guide**. Sports Illustrated.

Baum, Kenneth, and Trubo, Richard. **The Metal Edge: Maximize Your Sports Potential with the Mind/Body Connection**.

The Complete Guide to the Human Body. 2002. Noble Park, Victoria, Australia: Five Mile Press.

Dalgleish, J., and Dollery, S. 2001. **The Health and Fitness Handbook**. Essex: Pearson Education Limited.

Delavier, Frédérick. 2001. **Strength Training Anatomy**. Illinois: Human Kinetics.

Floyd, R.T., and Thompson, Clem W. 2003. **Manual of Structural Kinesiology** (14th ed.). McGraw-Hill Higher Education.

McCracken, Thomas, Gen. Ed. 2001. **New Atlas of Human Anatomy.** London: Constable.

Muybridge, Eadweard. 1955. **The Human Body in Motion.** New York: Dover Publications.

Steindler, Arthur. 1964. **Kinesiology of the Human Body.** Charles C. Thomas.

Sudy, Mitchell, Supervising Ed. 1991. **Personal Trainer Manual – The Resource for Fitness Instructors.** American Council on Exercise.

Viljoen, Wayne. 2003. **The Weight Training Handbook.** London: New Holland.

Wyatt, Tanya. (2004). **Be Your Own Personal Trainer.** London: New Holland.

WEBSITES

www.acefitness.org

www.acsm.org

www.anatomical.com

www.anatomy-resources.com

www.barmethod.com

www.barre3.com

www.basipilates.com

www.beachbody.com

www.beyondthewhiteboard.com

www.bodyworlds.com

www.bootcampmilitaryfitnessinstitute.com

www.crossfit.com

www.cyclebar.com

www.darebee.com

www.exrx.net

www.flywheelsports.com

www.ideafit.com

www.issaonline.edu

www.nsca.com

www.orangetheoryfitness.com

www.pelotoncycle.com

www.physique57.com

www.pilatesanytime.com

www.pilatesmethodalliance.org

www.ptonthenet.com

www.purebarre.com

www.robbwolf.com

www.scienceofrunning.com

www.soul-cycle.com

www.spinning.com

www.sport-fitness-advisor.com

www.stronglifts.com

www.toughmudder.com

www.trxtraining.com

www.webmd.com

www.womenfitness.net

www.yogaanytime.com

www.zonediet.com

www.zumba.com

www.zumbafitnessgame.com

Glossary

Abduction Movement of a limb away from the center line, such as lifting a straight arm laterally from one's side.

Adduction Movement of a limb toward the midline of the body, such as pulling a straight arm toward one's side.

AFAP CrossFit term meaning "as fast as possible."

Agonist A muscle that causes motion.

AMRAP CrossFit term meaning "as many reps/rounds as possible."

Anterior (ventral) The front of the body.

Antagonist A muscle that moves the joint opposite to the movement produced by the agonist.

Box CrossFit gym.

Circumduction Circular movement (combining flexion, extension, adduction, and abduction) with no shaft rotation.

Compound exercises Involving two or more joint movements.

Concentric A muscle contraction, resulting in its shortening.

Closed chain An exercise in which the end segment of the exercised limb is fixed, or supporting the weight. Most compound exercises are closed chain movements.

Cross-Fit Games The Superbowl of CrossFit.

Duration The number of sets or exercises for each specific muscle group. Duration may include number of repetitions.

Dynamic stabilizer A biarticulate muscle that simultaneously shortens at the target joint and lengthens the adjacent joint with no appreciable difference in length. Dynamic stabilization occurs during many compound movements.

Eccentric The contraction of a muscle during its lengthening.

EMOM CrossFit term meaning "every minute on the minute."

Eversion Moving the foot away from the medial plane.

Extension Straightening, extending, or opening out a joint, resulting in an increase of the angle between two bones.

External rotation Outward (lateral) rotation of a joint within the transverse plane of the body. The resulting movement will be toward the posterior (back) of the body.

Flexion Bending a joint, resulting in a decrease of angle.

For Time CrossFit term meaning that your goal is to finish the prescribed workout as quickly as you can.

Frequency The number of workouts per week (or unit time) or number of times a muscle group is trained per unit time.

Functional An exercise that allows one to gain motor development or strength in a manner in which it is used in the execution of a particular task (e.g., specific sport skill, occupational task, or daily activity).

HIIT High-intensity interval training.

Homeostasis The tendency of the body to maintain a stable equilibrium in physiological processes.

Hyperextension Extending a joint beyond its normal anatomical position.

Intensity The amount of weight used, percentage of one repetition maximum, or degree of effort used during exercise.

Internal rotation Inward medial rotation of a joint within the transverse plane of the body. Movement is directed toward the anterior (front) surface of the body.

Inversion Moving the sole of the foot toward the medial plane.

Isometric Contracting a muscle without significant movement; also referred to as static tension.

Lateral Away from sagittal midline of body.

Medial Toward sagittal midline of body.

Open chain An exercise in which the end segment of the exercised limb is not fixed, or is not supporting the weight. Most isolated exercises are open chain movements.

Paleo Caveman diet of animal protein, eggs, fruits, vegetables, mushrooms, nuts, seeds, herbs, and spices. Excludes dairy, grains, legumes, and processed food.

Posterior (dorsal) Located behind or to the back of the body.

Pronation Internal rotation of the foot or forearm.

ROM Range of motion. The amount of movement at each joint. Every joint in the body has a "normal" range of motion.

Rotation Circular (rotary) movement around the longitudinal axis of the bone.

Scaling Progression or regression of an exercise (i.e., making it easier or more difficult).

Synergist A muscle that assists another muscle to accomplish a movement.

Stabilizer A muscle that contracts with no significant movement.

Supination External rotation of the foot or forearm, resulting in an appendage facing upward.

Weight-bearing exercise Any type of activity that causes the body to react against gravity.

WOD CrossFit term meaning "workout of the day."

Index

NEW ANATOMY FOR STRENGTH AND FITNESS TRAINING

Additional Praise

"Contains a lot of good information... Well organized, easy to read, with clear pictures and text."

—Strength Basics blog

"A serious must-read for people interested in how their body's muscles and tendons work together to strengthen the body... a great addition to your fitness library."

—3 Fat Chicks On A Diet weight loss support website

"An excellent reference tool for understanding how specific exercises affect muscles and joints. Outstanding illustrations."

—Michael P. Garofalo, fitness trainer

"An excellent reference for those who wish to keep themselves fit. This book is a perfect guide for professional trainers as well as the one who works out at home."

—Health Over 50

"Vella's book makes my life so easy. It is clearly written, beautifully illustrated, very straight-forward, and will be at my side for the remainder of my professional career. It's not only a terrific reference for professionals, but I will be able to show my clients what's happening with their bodies—thereby making their workouts more effective. Absolutely indispensable book for anyone in the bodywork or body training field. Thank you, Mr. Vella."

—Charlotte, personal fitness trainer

"The one truism I have learned during many years of fitness training is that to continually improve you must never stop learning. **New Anatomy for Strength and Fitness Training** *is just that vehicle."*

—Cary Nosler, Host, Forever Young health radio talk show

About the Author

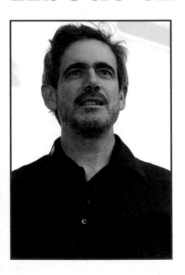

Born into an eclectic family surrounded by books and six spoken languages, Dr. Mark Vella, ND, developed a deep curiosity for learning and understanding the anatomy and physiology of life from an early age. He started his first personal training and lifestyle consultancy in 1991, paired with an extensive lecturing and course development career in the wellness and exercise sciences.

Having held multiple fitness qualifications, including American Council on Exercise and Exercise Teachers Academy, Mark furthered his studies into neuromuscular bodywork and Natural Medicine before advancing his professional practice towards mentoring individuals and organizations to exceptional performance at work, at home, and in life, guiding them to make better choices that produce real results. As a behavioral specialist drawing on his wellness and business background, his thought-leading work combines emotional intelligence, lifestyle medicine, governance principles, and entrepreneurial and strategic thinking.

Mark is registered as a Naturopathic Doctor with the Allied Health Professions Council of South Africa. He holds a Business Management Honors from The University of Cape Town Graduate School of Business. He has authored and designed over 30 wellness programs, courses, and qualifications, including the world's first Internet and call center protocol database in Natural Medicine. His books have sold over 180,000 copies and have been translated into nine languages.

With anatomy still a first love, his Training and Movement Anatomy Workshops draw on an integrated functional approach widely applicable to bodyworkers, personal trainers, coaches, and yoga teachers. In addition to his own workshops, Mark still lectures for the Body Arts and Science International (BASI). Further details can be found at *www.movementanatomy.com*. Further information on his mentorship practice can be found at *www.markvella.net*.